P9-DDW-670

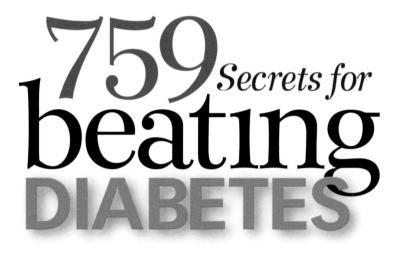

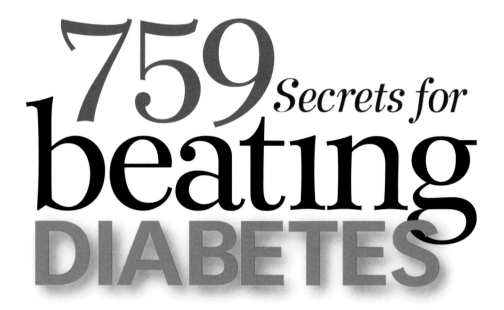

759 *Secrets for* beating DIABETES

simple, everyday tips to transform your health

Reader's Digest

The Reader's Digest Association, Inc.
Pleasantville, New York | Montreal

PROJECT STAFF

Editors
Marianne Wait,
Daryna Tobey

Cover Designer
Michele Laseau

Interior Designer
Rich Kershner

Writers
Jeff Bredenberg,
Marianne McGinnis,
Marie Suszynski

Advisor
Mary M. Austin, MA, RD, CDE

Recipe Developer
Robyn Webb, MS

Illustrators
exercises ©Shawn Banner,
cover, interior decorative
©Lyse-Anne Roy

Copy Editor
Marcia Mangum Cronin

Indexer
Cohen Carruth Indexes

READER'S DIGEST HOME & HEALTH BOOKS

President, Home & Garden and Health & Wellness
Alyce Alston

Editor in Chief
Neil Wertheimer

Creative Director
Michele Laseau

Executive Managing Editor
Donna Ruvituso

Associate Director, North America Prepress
Douglas A. Croll

Manufacturing Manager
John L. Cassidy

Marketing Director
Dawn Nelson

THE READER'S DIGEST ASSOCIATION, INC.

President and Chief Executive Officer
Mary Berner

President, Consumer Marketing
Dawn Zier

Copyright ©2007 by The Reader's Digest Association, Inc.
Copyright ©2007 by The Reader's Digest Association (Canada) ULC
Copyright ©2007 by The Reader's Digest Association Far East Ltd.
Philippine Copyright ©2007 by The Reader's Digest Association
Far East Ltd.

All rights reserved. Unauthorized reproduction, in any manner,
is prohibited.

Reader's Digest and the Pegasus logo are registered trademarks of
The Reader's Digest Association, Inc.

Library of Congress
Cataloging-in-Publication Data759 secrets for beating diabetes : simple,
everyday tips to transform your health.
    p. cm. – (Reader's Digest home & health books) Includes index.
ISBN 978-0-7621-0550-2 1.
Diabetes--Popular works. I. Title: Seven hundred fifty nine secrets for
beating diabetes.
RC660.4.A18 2007
616.4'62--dc22

                        2007042305

Address any comments about *759 Secrets for Beating Diabetes* to:

The Reader's Digest Association, Inc.
Editor in Chief, Home and Health Books
Reader's Digest Road
Pleasantville, NY 10570-7000

To order copies of *759 Secrets for Beating Diabetes,*
call 1-800-846-2100.
Visit our website at **rd.com**

Printed in the United States of America

5 7 9 10 8 6 4

US 6007/IC

Note to Readers

The information in this book should not be substituted for, or used to alter, medical therapy without your doctor's advice. For a specific health problem, consult your physician for guidance. The mention of any products, retail businesses, or Web sites in this book does not imply or constitute an endorsement by the authors or by the Reader's Digest Association, Inc.

Photo credits: page 31©David Bishop, page 42 courtesy Franklin Becker. Additional photography courtesy of Amana Images, Blend Images, BrandX, Comstock, Corbis, Creatas, Digital Vision, Fancy Photography, Foodcollection, Fstop, Getty Images, GoodShoot, The Image Bank, Image Source, Imagenavi, Johner Images, Jupiter Images, PhotoAlto, PhotoDisc, Photographer's Choice, Riser, StockByte, Vee

contents

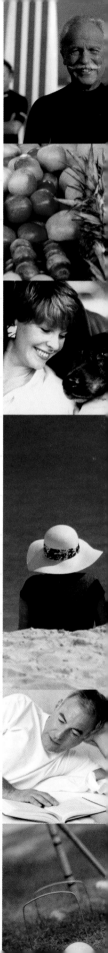

beat diabetes in every corner of your life

You do hundreds, even thousands, of things every day, from drinking your morning coffee to turning on the computer to humming a song. Many of them you don't even think about—they're just "what you do." Could some of them change a little without affecting your overall day? Certainly. And what if some of those changes offered the promise of significantly improving your health? Even better.

With that in mind, we've put together what may be the most comprehensive menu ever of small changes for better diabetes management. Each tip on the pages ahead is designed to help you feel great throughout the day, gain better control of your blood sugar, and protect your whole body from the damage that uncontrolled diabetes can cause.

Diabetes isn't a disease you leave at the doctor's office; you take it with you everywhere you go. On the plus side, you can fight it and improve your overall health, no matter where you are. We've created this book to help you beat your diabetes in every place in your life—your kitchen, your living room, your backyard, your neighborhood, your mind, and more. Because it's the little things you do, and think, between sunup and sundown that make the difference between beating this all-too-common disease and letting it beat you.

This book is mainly intended for people with type 2 diabetes. If you're reading it now, you're already ahead of the game because you're willing to try a few of our "simple, everyday tips to transform your health," as it says on the cover. These ideas truly are simple—some take mere minutes to execute—and you might even enjoy a few tiny changes in your routine, just as people enjoy writing with a new pen or wearing a new pair of shoes. If you follow even five or 10 of these clever suggestions regularly, you'll have made huge strides toward better health. Incorporate more over the course of time and you'll be surprised and delighted with what happens to your weight, your blood sugar levels, your energy, and your sense of well-being.

I should mention that just as you're different from everyone else, so is your diabetes different from everyone else's. These tips are appropriate for just about everyone, but work with your doctor and your registered dietitian to fit them into treatment plans and eating strategies that are exactly right for you. Here's to transforming your health, one easy step at a time.

Marianne Wait
Associate Editorial Director
Reader's Digest Books

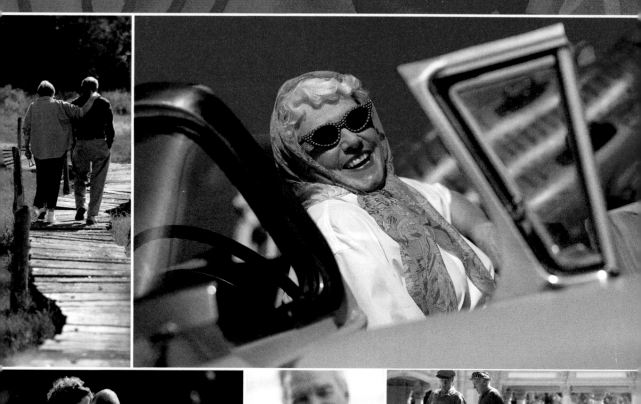

better-than-ever health

Welcome to the first day of a new beginning! You didn't ask
for a diabetes diagnosis, but it could be the ticket to a much
healthier, happier, energy-filled you.

a blessing in disguise

Most people with diabetes remember exactly when they were told they had it. It was likely a defining moment filled with all sorts of emotions, including fear. Fear, of course, is a natural reaction to learning you have a chronic disease. It's what you do with that fear that makes the difference. You can let it defeat you, and put yourself at the mercy of whatever may come, or you can use it to fight back and reclaim your health. This book is about fighting back in small, easy ways every day—and reaping more rewards than you can possibly imagine.

Some people say diabetes helped them "get their priorities straight."

Think of your type 2 diabetes diagnosis as a wake-up call, a request from your body to take better care of your health. That doesn't mean you *caused* your diabetes; genes play a strong role. But it does mean you need to start eating more nutritious foods in reasonable-size portions, exercising more, and even paying more attention to your stress levels and your nightly sleep habits. Diabetes isn't like a broken arm; you can't isolate the problem and let it heal while you go on with life as usual. Controlling it means taking steps that affect your whole body. And when you take them, your body, mind, and spirit will benefit.

In fact, some people who've managed their diabetes well say they are healthier now than they were before they were diagnosed; that the disease helped them "get their priorities straight." They have better habits and happier lives, and they're enjoying brighter moods, greater energy, and a stronger sense of personal control. You can, too, and it may take less effort than you think.

Have you noticed how giving a simple heartfelt compliment to your spouse once in a while can cut down on arguments? That putting all your new bills in one place is the trick to making sure they get paid? That having a stash of birthday cards on hand removes all panic when you remember a birthday at the last minute? Equally small measures can help you keep a better handle on your diabetes, and this book is chock-full of them. We'll walk you through tiny steps you can take in all the places you spend your time—and even in figurative "places" like your mind and your marriage—that will act like that compliment, that bill drawer, and that stack of birthday cards in heading off problems, helping you live smarter, and cutting down on unnecessary stress.

Let's be clear: It's your life to live, and these are your habits to adopt. Your doctor can't adopt them for you. He or she will give you exams, order lab tests, write prescriptions, and talk to you for several minutes per visit about how you're doing. But the truth about modern health care is this: The person in the white coat does not have time to oversee the management of your diabetes day in and day out. And you wouldn't really want your doctor in your kitchen (too many cooks!), in your car (backseat driver!), or at your desk at work (consider the terrible handwriting!). Your doc is an advisor who suggests a game plan. But you're the one who will carry it out, from the time you wake up and make the coffee and pour a *small* glass of orange juice to the time you snuggle yourself back into bed in time for a full night's sleep.

That doesn't mean you have to go it alone. In fact, you'll want and need plenty of people in your corner, from your MD to a registered dietitian (RD) and maybe a certified diabetes educator (CDE) and/or a diabetes support group. You'll read more about each of these resources later in the book. But at the center of this health-care team is one person: you. So seek every bit of help you can get in terms of professional guidance and advice—then be prepared to take matters into your own hands. The sooner the better. The fact is, most people with diabetes had it for several years before they were diagnosed. And diabetes is a progressive disease; it tends to get worse over time. But with this book in hand, and more than 700 simple, clever tips at your disposal, you can get the better of it—and love your life like never before.

diabetes: an exceptional disease

With most diseases, it's fairly easy to picture what's wrong and how to fix it. If you have cancer, you cut it out, or bomb it with radiation. If your arteries are clogged, you cut out the steak and sour cream. Diabetes is different. The problems involved—at the core, an inability to produce and/or use enough of the hormone insulin to process the glucose, or blood sugar, that fuels your cells—are hard to visualize, which may make the disease seem less "real." But it's real all right. And the "simple" problem of high blood sugar doesn't end with your blood. Diabetes has a cascade of effects, damaging a number of body systems as it progresses.

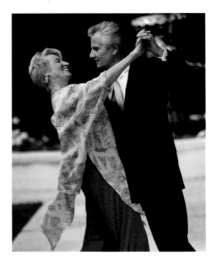

For the rest of your life, your diabetes is going to be somewhere along a continuum: At the early stages, there are typically few symptoms or complications—you'll actually be a relatively healthy person. At the opposite end of the continuum are the serious complications that result when this chronic disease goes unchecked—blindness, kidney disease, amputation, nerve damage, sexual dysfunction, and heart disease, for instance. Among people with diabetes, 65 percent die of heart disease or stroke. Diabetes causes 44 percent of all cases of kidney failure, and 60 to 70 percent of people with diabetes have some degree of nerve damage. Men who have diabetes are twice as likely to have erectile dysfunction as men who don't have diabetes.

Those figures are sobering indeed. But here's the silver lining: You can stop or slow your progress along that continuum at any time. You may even be able to go backward. And it won't take a miracle, just plain old determination and persistence.

top habits to adopt

A diabetes diagnosis often brings with it a mind-numbing barrage of medication regimens, testing schedules, meal plans, and more. For goodness' sake, even if you didn't have high blood pressure before, you do now! Frustration levels run so high among patients, it's no wonder that "diabetes burnout" (frazzled patients on the brink of giving up) is a major concern in the medical community. Some people get so overwhelmed that they throw in the towel and revert to their old habits.

Can You "Beat" Diabetes?

We say yes. It's true that there's currently no cure for the disease. But you can reverse both of the core problems—insulin resistance and lack of insulin secretion—by tweaking what you eat and how often you exercise. Long term, if you're serious about making changes to the way you live every day, you could possibly even reduce your need for medication or insulin.

You'll see results right away when you start following the advice in this book. In fact, you could see positive blood-sugar changes from some of the tips in a matter or days or even hours. Over time, making some of our strategies part of your daily routine could make the difference between, say, losing your sight or not.

Your efforts to beat your diabetes will have a profound effect. For instance, researchers say that for every one-point drop in your A1C blood sugar score (a measure of blood sugar over the last three months), you reduce your odds of eye, kidney, and nerve damage by 40 percent. Controlling your blood pressure when you have diabetes can reduce your risk of heart disease by as much as 50 percent and your risk of eye damage by 33 percent. Foot care programs for people with diabetes are known to reduce rates of amputation by 45 to 85 percent. With results like that within your power, there's just no reason to sit back and do nothing.

In a way, this book is all about battling burnout. The tips are useful, easy, and even fun, and there are plenty that you've never heard before. You don't have to follow them all, just choose a few to start with—maybe adding an extra vegetable serving at dinner and a short walk after your meal—then dip back into the book and add a few more when you're ready. They'll make a noticeable difference before you know it.

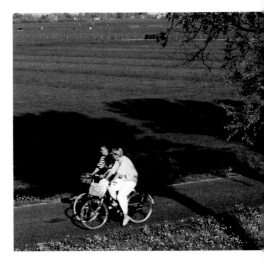

Many of our everyday "secrets" are designed to help you do the things that matter most to your diabetes. For instance, many studies show that losing just 5 to 7 percent of your body weight—that's about 10 pounds if you weigh 160 pounds—can reduce your insulin resistance, increase your insulin secretion, and lower your blood sugar levels, essentially putting the disease in reverse. Here are some of the most important overall goals we'll help you accomplish. Of course it's also absolutely critical to take any medications your doctor has prescribed, on time and without fail.

Monitor Your Blood Sugar

There's an old saying among people who study management: "That which gets measured gets done." Translation? You are much more likely to achieve goals if you are getting constant feedback that documents the results of your efforts. In controlling diabetes, this means checking the glucose levels in a drop of your blood—possibly several times a day, depending upon your situation. The results show you how your body is reacting to the foods you eat, the medications you take, the exercise you get, and even the stress you're under. Manufacturers are bending over backward to make testing as convenient and pain-free as possible, so stay alert to innovations in testing technology.

Keep Calories Under Control

You will hear a lot of talk about sugar and carbohydrates as they pertain to diabetes, but the ultimate goal for most people is to reduce calorie consumption to a level that allows you to gradually lose weight. The most powerful way to do this and to get the nutrition your body needs is to emphasize fruits, vegetables, and whole grains, while cutting back on red meat, ice cream, cookies, and junk food. Of course, watching your portion sizes is also critical. Excess body fat is the most significant factor in the development of type 2 diabetes, and losing weight is priority number 1 if you want to control the disease.

Eat Smarter Carbs

It's important to control the amount of carbohydrate you eat, since it's mainly carbohydrate foods that raise blood sugar, and you'll discover tips for finding and reaching your daily carbohydrate targets in this book. But changing the *type* of carbohydrates you eat might be every bit as important, since some carb foods raise blood sugar higher and faster than others. Eating lower on the glycemic index—something you'll read about later on—has emerged as a critical step in keeping weight and blood sugar under control. It means switching to foods made from whole grains (like whole-wheat bread, old-fashioned oatmeal, and barley side dishes) and cutting down on foods made from white flour (think white bread and bagels) as well as other refined grains, such as white rice. It also means cutting down on foods made from grains that have been processed to the point where they're practically predigested (like whole-wheat breads that have the same look, feel, and texture as white bread) and scaling back on very starchy foods such as rice and potatoes, as well as on soda and other sugary drinks.

Get Off the Couch

We are in the midst of an epidemic of "sitting disease." Most of us move through a daily progression of sitting in the car, then sitting at our desks, then sitting in the car again, then sitting on the couch. All this sitting contributes to a widening waistline, and experts blame obesity as one of the main factors fueling the current explosion of diabetes cases.

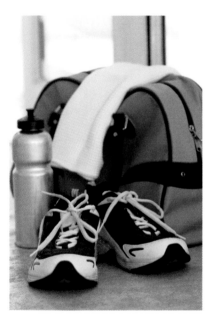

Exercise is one of the most important things you can do for your body, your mind, and your diabetes. When you move your body more, you burn more calories. You also build muscle, which boosts your metabolism. It's possible to lose weight through diet alone, but it's much easier when you combine calorie cutting with physical activity. Ideally, use a blend of aerobic exercise (walking, swimming, cycling, and other heart-pumping activities) with strength training (weight lifting and calisthenics, for instance).

Exercise does more than help you lose weight. Losing fat and increasing muscle makes cells more sensitive to insulin so they can take up more glucose and leave your blood sugar levels lower. That's why following a healthful diet and increasing physical activity are two of the most powerful tools in preventing or controlling type 2 diabetes.

Keep Your Blood Sugar and Blood Pressure in the "Zone"

Much of diabetes control focuses on keeping blood sugar as near as possible to the normal range. That's because this strategy has been proven to prevent damage to the eyes, kidneys, and nerves—common complications of diabetes. Certain other health problems often accompany high blood sugar, including high blood pressure, high cholesterol, and high triglycerides, which all contribute to heart disease. In fact, high blood pressure does more harm to your heart than the high blood sugar does. Conveniently, the same strategies that help to control your blood sugar, such as moderate exercise, healthy eating, and weight loss, will also do a world of good for the health of your heart.

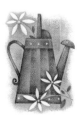

You are the "hub" of your disease management team.

Get Support

If you've been reluctant in the past to interact with doctors and other medical professionals, get over it. You need ongoing relationships with the experts who can regularly evaluate aspects of your health, answer your questions, and provide the tools and medications you need to control your diabetes. These professionals would typically include a doctor who specializes in diabetes, a diabetes educator who can give you the one-on-one coaching that your doctor doesn't have time for, and a registered dietitian who will help you establish a way of eating that's based on your goals and your tastes. You also will need an eye doctor, a foot doctor, and a dentist. Find a good pharmacist who will give you pointers on medications. A mental health professional can give valuable advice for coping with the emotional issues that many diabetes patients face.

Keep the Information Flowing

The term "health care team" evokes the image of a doctor, an endocrinologist, a nurse, and a dietitian all wearing T-shirts emblazoned with your name and huddling every morning to mull over your lab reports. Well, you may very well attend a health center that has a "team" approach in place, but you can't assume that your case is getting such a high level of scrutiny or that your health care professionals are even trading data about you very efficiently. It's likely that the professionals you recruit to make up your health care team are not even acquainted with one another and swap only minimal information about your case—if any at all. *You* are the "hub" of your disease management team, and it's up to you to make sure that all the members are up to date. (Hint: You'll need to keep good records, bring them with you to appointments, and learn to speak up.)

are you ready?

When you catch a cold, it will go away after a week or two. Having diabetes is not like that. Unfortunately, your diabetes will never go away. It's there, even if you'd prefer to ignore it, and if you ignore it, it will get worse. On the other hand, if you accept the fact that diabetes is part of your life and decide to fight back, you can slash your risk of diabetes-related health problems just by adopting a few new habits here and there that will make you feel better no matter what motivated you to try them. And when you feel good, you'll have the motivation and energy you need to implement a few more changes.

Before you know it, you'll start to really appreciate the taste, tang, crunch, zing, and texture of fresh whole foods; you'll savor the 30 minutes in your day that you reserve for a mind-cleansing, stress-relieving walk; you'll feel stronger; your clothes will fit better; and you'll wake up in the morning with a more positive attitude. If you have to have diabetes, why not use it as an excuse to lead a healthier, more enjoyable life? We've given you more than 700 ways to do it. Pick one and start today.

chapter one

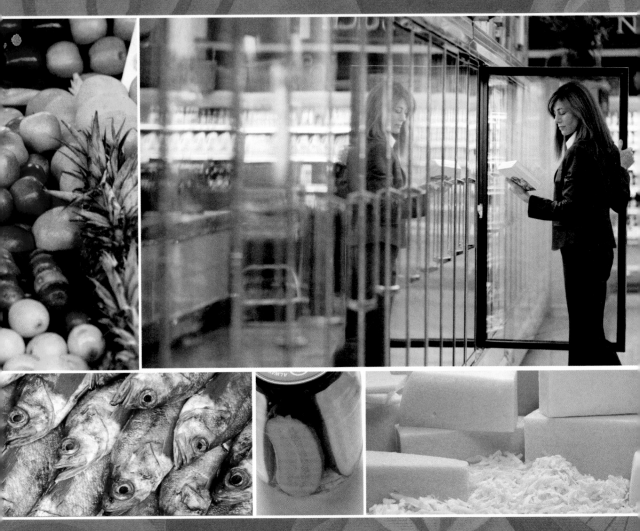

at the grocery store

Walk into these lands of plenty armed with a plan.
Because how you shop dictates how well you eat at home—and
how well you manage your diabetes.

walk in with a plan

The most successful shopping trip starts before you even head out the door. That's because knowing what to buy means first knowing what you're going to eat! Job one, then, is doing a bit of advance planning on the menu front. You'll also want to follow some of our smarter-shopping tips to help you better control the foods that you allow into your home.

Shop with a detailed list in hand and check off items as you shop. In the next chapter you'll read how important it is to plan your meals and get some tips for doing it. Make a shopping list based on the meals you've planned, and don't buy anything that isn't on the list, except for staples such as toilet paper and laundry detergent. With your list firmly in hand, you'll find no excuse to throw junk food into your cart. By the way, studies show that people who plan their meals and make detailed shopping lists eat more vegetables than those who don't. Check off the items as you shop so you won't go home missing an ingredient.

Take a mental stroll around the grocery store before you put pen to paper. If you go to the same grocery store every week, you probably know the layout like the back of your hand. As you make out your shopping list, think about the path you take when you're navigating the aisles, and write your list out in that order. This way, you'll never have to backtrack through any department, helping you avoid those impulse buys like the chips you couldn't resist the third time you passed them. This also will allow you to plot a strategy for avoiding the aisles that tempt you most (did someone say ice cream?).

Plan to spend most of your time around the perimeter of the store. This, after all, is where you'll find the fresh, whole foods—the produce, the

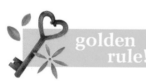

golden rule! **Buy Food Your Grandma Would Have Recognized**

Chances are, Grandma in her shopping days never laid eyes on candy-colored fruit snacks, granola bars laden with chocolate and marshmallows, or frozen French toast. But she certainly would have recognized fresh fruits and vegetables, meats and poultry, fish, and other "whole" foods in their natural state. So buy bananas instead of banana-flavored pud-

ding, pork cutlets over hot dogs, and fresh or bagged spinach over spinach in a box that comes with its own fat-laden, over-salted sauce. Not only will you maximize your vitamin and mineral intake, you won't ingest the sodium, sugar, processed fats, and chemical additives that are found in so many processed foods.

yogurt, the chicken, the fish. Of course, you'll need to venture into the belly of the store for your olive oil, your canned tomatoes and beans, and your whole grains and cereals. But fresh foods, especially fruits and vegetables, should take up the bulk of your shopping cart.

Do your nutritional sleuthing on the Web. The supermarket isn't a library—you don't have to spend your time at the store squinting at food labels. If you have an Internet connection, you can do all the nutritional research you want at home before you go shopping. A Web site called Nutrition Data (www.nutritiondata.com) lists the facts on the calories, fat, cholesterol, and carbohydrates in many of the foods—from chocolate bars and boxed cereals to apples and kidney beans—you'll find in the grocery store. This is an especially helpful tool if you're counting carbohydrates for blood sugar control. (See chapter two for a primer on carbohydrate counting.)

Eat a healthy snack before you leave the house. If your stomach is growling while you shop, you're more likely to come home with precisely what you *shouldn't* be eating: convenience foods in boxes and packages that are high in sugar, fat, or salt—or all three! And if you've just eaten a fresh summer peach before you get to the grocery store, it'll remind you to buy more of them while you're there.

Don't be afraid to pay more for fresh foods. Rest assured, your food budget will even out in the end because of the things you're *not* buying— namely, junk food. A 12-ounce bag of chips can cost $3.99, which adds up to more than $5 a pound—much more than a pound of apples or bananas costs. And a bag of dry beans or barley is practically a give-away and will last you for weeks, compared to an over-priced (and undernourished) frozen dinner, which will be gone in a day. Lastly, keep this in mind: By eating better today, you may one day be able to better control your blood sugar and possibly cut down on your diabetes medications—and pay less at the pharmacy.

Rate yourself when you get home. Look at your receipt and highlight all of your healthful food purchases: fresh and frozen fruits and vegetables, whole grains, low-fat dairy foods, dried or low-sodium canned beans and peas, lean meats, fish, nuts, and olive oil. Most of your receipt should be highlighted, with only a few lines of indulgent snacks and ready-made foods left out. Use this list as a starting point for an even healthier grocery trip next week.

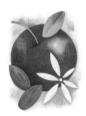

By eating better, you may be able to cut down on your medications and pay less at the pharmacy.

linger in the produce department

It's no wonder that restaurants garnish their plates with parsley, tomato wedges, and cleverly carved radishes—vegetables' vibrant colors and unexpected textures infuse pizzazz into every meal. But what's more important is the nutritional benefit that vegetables offer: They're chock-full of fiber, vitamins, and disease-fighting antioxidants, and they're generally low in both calories and carbohydrates. If there's anywhere in the supermarket that you should allow yourself to make impulse purchases, it's here.

Designate a veggie of the week. Tired of the same old tomatoes and corn? Good! It's time to try something new, especially if a little variety helps you eat more vegetables. To sneak in an extra serving of vegetables every day, buy a vegetable you've never tried—or one that you haven't eaten in a long time—and then challenge yourself to work it into your diet every day that week. It could be as simple as broccoli or green beans or as exotic as bok choy. Your goal: Have none of it left to throw out at the end of the week.

Take the free recipe. Many supermarkets give away recipes that spotlight fresh vegetables in an effort to get customers to eat (and buy) more produce. Usually the featured recipes are for in-season, sometimes exotic veggies. Take one and give it a try!

Darken your greens. It's smart to shake yourself out of the iceberg lettuce habit. Not only do baby spinach, arugula, watercress, and green lettuces (Romaine, green leaf, Boston, and Bibb) bring new crunch and flavor to your salads, they also pack in more vitamins. For example, a cup of iceberg lettuce contains 7 percent of your daily vitamin A needs; a cup of raw spinach leaves is packed with more than 50 percent, plus 14 percent of your vitamin C needs.

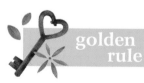

golden rule!   ## Fill Up to Half of Your Cart with Colorful Produce

Those colors indicate the presence of different phytochemicals including antioxidants, which work together to neutralize free radicals, harmful molecules that your body may have in excess if you have diabetes. These free radicals wreak havoc on cells and can increase your chances of suffering diabetes-related complications as well as heart disease. The deeper or more intense the color of the produce, the better. See red with tomatoes and red bell peppers, opt for orange with carrots, mangoes, or cantaloupe, and go green with broccoli, kale, and spinach. Your meals will look and taste more interesting to boot.

whip it together! Broccoli Surprise Salad

Broccoli and strawberries join together in this palate-pleasing salad packed with vitamins, fiber—and flavor!

In a bowl, mix together 2 cups of fresh **broccoli florets**, ½ cup of quartered **strawberries**, 2 tablespoons of sliced **almonds** or roasted **flaxseeds** (that's 6 additional grams of fiber!), and 1 ounce of shredded reduced-fat sharp **cheddar cheese**. Prepare the dressing in a smaller bowl by mixing ¼ cup reduced-fat **mayonnaise**, ½ tablespoon of **sugar** or **sugar substitute**, and 1 teaspoon **cider vinegar**. Pour over the salad and mix well.

Splurge on prewashed, precut veggies. Yes, a bag of prewashed spinach is more expensive than a bunch of regular spinach, and the same goes for precut carrots, celery, and peppers versus veggies you have to peel, wash, and slice yourself. But the investment can be well worth it if you're pressed for time, or if the prep work discourages you from eating veggies at all.

Buy enough fruits and vegetables to get you through the week. That means three to five days' worth of fresh produce, supplemented with frozen or canned. "I haven't gone to the store in a week" is no excuse not to get at least five servings of vegetables per day. Frozen vegetables contain as many nutrients as their fresh counterparts—and they're easy to use. Sneaking a serving of frozen corn into your chili, or two servings of frozen spinach into lasagna or tuna casserole, are simple ways to ramp up your veggie intake.

Make your own veggie ice cubes. Frozen onions are convenient—but expensive. Instead, chop items such as onions, celery, carrots, parsley, or garlic, fill a plastic ice cube tray with them, add a little water (broth won't work), then freeze. Once they're frozen, put the cubes in a labeled plastic freezer bag or plastic box in the freezer. Add a cube or two to recipes as needed. This is also a good way to save produce that you can't use in time.

Mix and match your produce. Fruits and vegetables suddenly become more interesting when you eat them in unexpected combinations. Try shredded carrots paired with chopped mangos, or pineapple paired with red onions, as toppings for grilled chicken breasts. Even cauliflower and green grapes pair well to make a crunchy, tangy salad. Simply wash a head of cauliflower and break it into bit-size pieces. Toss it with a cup of halved green grapes and a cup of toasted and coarsely chopped walnuts. Then add a dressing made by mixing ½ cup fat-free or light mayonnaise, ¼ cup honey, and 1 tablespoon yellow mustard. You'll have enough for at least 10 servings.

get your fill of fruit

Bananas on your cereal. Strawberry shortcake. Lip-smacking apple slices dipped in peanut butter. With treats as sweet as these, why do we grumble and groan when the doctor reminds us to eat more fruit? It's a gold mine for the vitamins and minerals your body needs including vitamin C, which helps prevent the damage that high blood sugar does to cells and arteries.

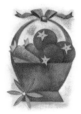

Cantaloupe is rich in vitamin A. It protects against some of diabetes' major complications.

Squeeze more citrus fruit into your cart. Oranges, lemons, limes, and grapefruit aren't just rich in vitamin C, they're surprisingly good sources of fiber. (One large orange contains 4 grams.) Lemon and lime juice are delicious in homemade salad dressings. The zest can be grated into vinaigrette dressings or added to the dry ingredients of breads and cakes. Lemons may have another advantage: Some preliminary research suggests that acidic foods like lemon actually blunt the effect of meals on your blood sugar. Buy a few extra lemons and plan to add the juice to everything from tuna sandwiches to pasta dishes.

Bag some apples. Want to keep your blood sugar on an even keel? Heed the old saying about eating apples to keep the doctor away. Apples are loaded with soluble fiber, which slows the digestion of food and thus the entry of glucose into the bloodstream. One group of researchers discovered that women who ate at least one apple a day were 28 percent less likely to develop diabetes than those who ate none. Apples are also rich in flavonoids, antioxidants that help prevent heart disease—if you eat the skin.

Put a cantaloupe in your cart. These melons are real standouts in the vitamin C department. And despite their sweetness, melons don't contain a lot of sugar, so forget anything you've heard about banning them from your diet. Can't use up a whole cantaloupe by having a slice every morning with breakfast? No problem. Cut it into chunks and scatter them in some sugar-free flavored gelatin, then chill. Voila—an easy, low-fat dessert. A cup of melon contains more than your recommended daily allowance of vitamin A, essential protection against some of diabetes' major complications, such as kidney and retina problems.

Buy as many berries as you can eat in a week. They may be candy to your taste buds, but their sweetness is deceptive. Fructose, the natural sugar found in most fruits, is sweeter than sucrose (table sugar), so it takes much less (with fewer calories) to get that sweet taste. And fructose is friendlier to blood sugar, causing a much slower rise than sucrose does. Berries are chock-full of fiber, not to mention anthocyanins, healthful plant compounds that scientists believe may help lower blood sugar by boosting insulin production.

fill your cart with smarter carbs

Carbohydrates aren't the devil, despite their reputation. Yes, they do raise blood sugar. But cutting them out isn't the answer, for many good reasons. The trick is controlling the types of carbs you eat and how much of them you consume. You'll definitely want to up your intake of whole grains, not only for their fiber but also for their antioxidants, vitamins, and minerals.

Choose cereal with at least 5 grams of fiber per serving. Among other benefits, fiber helps you feel full so you can get through the morning with only a small snack, if anything, before lunch. Fiber from bran cereal is also associated with less inflammation in women with type 2 diabetes. That's important because experts believe inflammation plays a major role in diabetes as well as the development of heart disease. The Physicians' Health Study found that doctors who ate whole-grain cereal every day were 28 percent less likely to have heart failure over 24 years.

Buy old-fashioned oats instead of instant-cereal packets. If you're debating between oatmeal and cold cereal, choose oatmeal. It has fewer calories than most cold cereals, and, unlike most cold cereals, oatmeal is high in sugar-stabilizing soluble fiber. In fact, research has found that eating one cup of oatmeal five or six times a week can reduce the risk of getting type 2 diabetes by 39 percent. It also helps lower cholesterol. But the instant breakfast packets usually contain added sugar, not to mention sodium, which can raise blood pressure. Apple-flavored instant oatmeal from a packet has 229 milligrams of sodium. A cup of rolled oats has only 3 milligrams of sodium—and its hearty, chewy texture just can't be beat.

Choose bread with the word "whole" in the first ingredient. Looking at the bread's color won't tell you if it's really whole grain—you have to read the ingredients list. Breads that list "enriched wheat flour" as the

---

whip it together!   Barley and Chickpea Salad

Don't shy away from buying barley just because you don't know what to do with it. This delicious, fiber-rich salad is easy to throw together from shelf staples.

Cook ⅔ cup **barley** according to the package directions, then let it cool for about half an hour. In a bowl, combine the cooked barley with 1 can (15 ounces) of drained and rinsed **chickpeas**, 10 sliced rehydrated **sun-dried tomatoes**, 1 can (15 ounces) **artichokes** packed in water, drained and halved, 3 minced **scallions**, and 2 minced **garlic** cloves. Mix well. Toss with ½ cup fat-free **Italian salad dressing**.

primary ingredient have been stripped of most of their nutrients—in fact, about 11 vitamins and minerals are lost in the process. Breads that are enriched also contain added sugar and fat.

Embrace chewy, dense loaves with visible kernels. Even if you choose a bread that's 100 percent whole wheat, it may not be as friendly to your blood sugar as it could be. If the wheat has been finely ground to the point that the bread has the texture of white bread, it will be digested nearly as fast as white bread and have similar effects on your blood sugar. Coarser grains take longer to digest and will raise blood sugar more slowly. Health-food stores will have this kind of bread if your local supermarket does not.

Look for extra-fiber breads. Some companies are selling bread with increased fiber and fewer carbs; two slices contain the same amount of carbohydrates that are in one slice of regular bread. You can also find English muffins that have 8 grams of fiber per serving for 100 calories—that's 35 percent of your daily fiber target. Consuming 25 grams of fiber a day helps lower cholesterol and control blood sugar levels.

Bulk up your stock of canned beans and lentils. These are "complex carbs" that also supply a load of protein without a lot of calories or fat, making them nearly perfect foods. Keep black beans, kidney beans, pinto beans, chickpeas, white beans, and lentils on hand to add to your soups, salads, and pasta dishes. Tossing just half a cup of canned chickpeas into tonight's salad will add 6 grams of fiber and 6 grams of protein.

Upgrade your pasta to whole wheat. You might think there's nothing worse for your blood sugar than pasta, but thanks to the durum wheat it's made from and the structure of the protein in pasta dough, that's not true. As it turns out, pasta has only a moderate effect on blood sugar levels— much more modest than that of the white Italian bread you might eat with

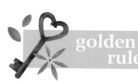

golden rule!   Aim to Eat Three Servings of Whole Grains a Day

Studies show that the more whole grains people eat, the greater their sensitivity to insulin and the lower their risk of developing diabetes. What's more, according to a study by researchers at the Wake Forest University School of Medicine, consuming just two and a half servings of whole grains per day is associated with a 21 percent lower risk of cardiovascular disease compared to consuming only 0.2 servings. What counts as a serving? One small slice of 100 percent whole-wheat bread, one-half cup of cooked oatmeal, or about three-quarters cup of whole-grain cereal.

whip it together! Spinach and Cannellini Bean Linguine

Make whole-wheat pasta interesting—and add lots of fiber and nutrients—with this hearty, quick-to-fix dish. Canned salmon boosts the protein and provides heart-healthy omega-3 fatty acids.

Bring a pot of water to boil, **salt** lightly. Add 1 pound of **whole-wheat linguine** and cook for 7 minutes or until al dente. As the pasta cooks, heat 1 tablespoon **olive oil** in a skillet. Sauté three minced **garlic** cloves in the oil for 30 seconds. Add 2 cups bagged **baby spinach leaves** and sauté for 1 to 2 minutes. Add in 1 cup canned, drained, and rinsed **cannellini beans** and 1 cup water-packed, reduced-sodium, **canned flaked salmon**. Drain the pasta, reserving about ⅓ cup of the cooking water. Add the cooking water to the spinach-garlic-bean mixture and mix. Add the sauce to the pasta and toss well. Season with **salt** and **pepper**.

your meal. But you'll get about three times the fiber per serving if you choose whole wheat. Not all brands and shapes taste as good in whole wheat; experiment to find one you like.

Also look for powered-up pastas. They contain extra protein and even more fiber. Some are made from grains such as oats, spelt, and barley, in addition to durum wheat, and since these grains are higher in soluble fiber than wheat, these pastas should be friendlier to your blood sugar.

Reach for brown rice instead of white. White rice is a refined carbohydrate, which will quickly convert to glucose in the body and send your blood sugar soaring. Brown rice, on the other hand, is a whole grain; a cup of cooked brown rice has 4 grams of fiber, compared to just 1 gram in white rice. Even brown rice raises blood sugar more than oatmeal or barley, but still, it offers the benefits of a whole-grain food.

When you don't want brown rice, choose converted rice. The rice is steamed before it's husked, allowing the individual grains to absorb more nutrients. It raises blood sugar slightly less than brown rice does, though it doesn't contain as much good-for-you fiber or as many nutrients as brown rice does.

Buy a bag of barley. One of the most underappreciated cereal grains, barley can be used instead of rice or noodles in soups, stews, and bean salads. Thanks to its impressive stash of soluble fiber, which slows the digestion of food and therefore the rise of blood sugar, it's much friendlier to blood sugar than rice for most people. And it lowers cholesterol to boot.

dial up your dairy intake

Many of us haven't downed a glass of milk since we were kids. We get our milk in dribs and drabs by adding it to coffee, cereal, and tea. But eating more dairy foods is one of the smartest things you can do to combat diabetes. Two Harvard studies found that people who made dairy foods part of their daily diets were 21 percent less likely to develop insulin resistance and 9 percent less likely to develop type 2 diabetes. And research has found that the more calcium and vitamin D people get in their diets, the less likely they are to develop metabolic syndrome, which ups the risk for heart disease. Diary foods may even help you shed spare pounds—which helps your body respond better to insulin and makes blood sugar control easier. Finally, low-fat dairy foods are a cornerstone of the DASH diet, designed to lower high blood pressure.

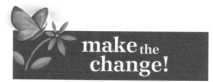

make the change!

The habit: Getting at least four servings of calcium-rich foods a day.

The result: Potentially lowering your risk of developing metabolic syndrome, heart disease, and other diabetes complications by about a third.

The proof: Researchers studied the diets of 80,000 women in the Nurses' Health Study for more than 20 years and found that those who got more than 1,200 milligrams of calcium and more than 800 international units of vitamin D a day had a 33 percent lower risk of developing type 2 diabetes compared with women who got less. In another study of more than 10,000 women age 45 and older, getting more calcium and vitamin D lowered the risk of having metabolic syndrome, a cluster of symptoms that can lead to type 2 diabetes and heart disease. Women with a higher calcium intake also had lower cholesterol. An 8-ounce glass of milk contains about 300 milligrams of calcium—just choose the fat-free and 1 percent fat varieties to curtail your intake of saturated fats.

Choose skim milk. Yes, whole milk tastes richer and creamier, but one cup contains 24 grams of cholesterol and 8 grams of fat—5 of them saturated fat. A cup of fat-free milk will give you all of the calcium and vitamin D of the whole milk while saving you 60 calories and all of the fat.

To wean yourself off fatty milk, buy milk that's one step down in fat. Switching from whole milk to skim in one shot will be a big shock to your taste buds. Instead, first make the switch from whole milk to 2 percent milk. When your 2 percent milk is half gone, fill the container back up with 1 percent milk. From 1 percent, the switch to skim is not such a shock. (Some stores even stock half-percent milk for an added step before you go completely fat-free.)

Buy some powdered skim milk. Stir a little into your glass of fat-free milk to power it up with more body and richness.

Keep a can of evaporated skim milk on hand. It doesn't contain any saturated fat, so it's perfect for adding to coffee or using in recipes that call for cream. It even makes a great gravy: Roast carrots, celery, and onions and mash them. Then add a bit of flour to the pan and cook to make a roux. Put the mixture in a blender with a little evaporated skim milk, and reheat the mixture on the stove.

Use evaporated milk to whip up a sweet topping. Instead of using whipped cream, pour in some reduced-fat evaporated milk, then add Splenda or another sweetener to taste. Grab a whisk, and whip away! (This is one case in which we'd advise against fat-free evaporated milk—it just doesn't whip as well.)

Choose nonfat, unsweetened (plain) yogurt and add your own mix-ins. This gives you the dual benefit of avoiding the saturated fat in whole-milk yogurt and avoiding the extra sugar in sweetened yogurt. If you add, say, a cup of fresh strawberries to plain yogurt, you can add 3 grams of fiber and plenty of natural fruit sweetness. For crunch, add some low-fat granola, bran cereal, or ground flaxseeds.

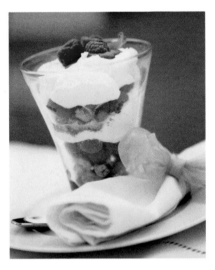

Purchase low-fat cheese—selectively. Let's face it— some low-fat cheeses just aren't worth eating. But if you're using, say, Monterey Jack or cheddar in casseroles or on top of chili, the low-fat versions will work just fine, and you won't really notice the difference. Using low-fat cheddar instead of regular will save you about 65 calories and 5 grams of saturated fat per ounce. This small switch goes a long way to cutting cholesterol and lowering your risk for heart disease.

Look sharp when it comes to cheese. Here's a secret trick that gourmet chefs use all the time: Pick out a very flavorful, pungent cheese—like extra-sharp cheddar, Romano, or Parmigiano-Reggiano—and only use a little of it on top of pastas or salads. This trick will not sacrifice flavor, but it will save you money (the less you use, the more money you save) as well as artery-clogging saturated fat (since you'll be using less of it).

Throw a carton of soy milk into your cart. Soy milk, tofu, and other soy products are good sources of calcium. What's more, soy protein has been shown to lower protein levels in the urine of type 2 diabetics (a sign of better kidney function) while slightly improving levels of HDL or "good" cholesterol. In one study involving overweight people who drank either dairy-based or soy-based meal replacement drinks, the soy group saw their blood sugar drop. Soy has also been shown to reduce the risk of some cancers. Avoid flavored soy milks, though, which contain added sugar. Soy milk will last for about a week in the fridge after you open it.

load up on lean protein

Protein has little or no effect on your blood sugar, so every time you mix some protein into your meals (and subtract some carbs), you automatically lower the blood sugar impact of your meal. Protein also helps keep hunger at bay between meals, facilitating weight loss. That said, there's no call to go overboard. Some doctors warn against consuming too much protein if you have diabetes because of the strain it puts on the kidneys (many people with diabetes are at high risk for kidney disease). And the saturated fat in red meat contributes to insulin resistance. The trick then, is to choose lean protein, and fortunately, that's a relatively easy feat.

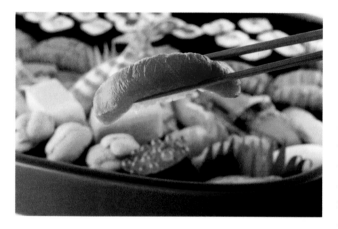

Head to the sushi station for a protein-packed prepared meal. Many larger supermarkets have their very own sushi chefs on-site, boxing up fresh fish and rice combination plates. If ever you need a quick, prepackaged meal, this is the place to stop: Sushi delivers protein and some fiber and is generally low in calories—one piece of a California roll has just 30 calories and less than a gram of fat. Just steer clear of the soy sauce, which is very high in sodium, or ask for the low-sodium kind.

Don't forget the eggs. Eggs have been much maligned over the years, but the fact is, they are an excellent and inexpensive source of protein and the most nutritionally complete of all protein sources. One large, hard-boiled egg contains 7 grams of protein and has just 2 grams of saturated fat. To avoid the saturated fat altogether, use the egg whites and throw out the yolks. Or you can dress that egg up (and get in a serving of veggies) by making an omelet and folding in iron- and fiber-rich spinach. In studies, people who ate eggs and toast for breakfast stayed full longer and ate significantly fewer calories the rest of the day than people who ate a bagel and cream cheese. Eggs do contain a fair amount of cholesterol, but dozens of studies have shown that it's saturated fat, not dietary cholesterol, that raises people's cholesterol the most.

Go for ground sirloin, the leanest ground beef. A 3-ounce serving has 196 calories and 10 grams of fat. The next leanest is ground round (for 218 calories, 13 grams of fat), then ground chuck and ground beef (both about 231 calories, 15 grams of fat).

Buy at most two servings of red meat per person per week. Red meat contains saturated fat, and one study found that women with type 2 diabetes who ate more red meat were more likely to develop heart disease than women with diabetes who ate less. Other research showed that the more red meat women ate over almost nine years, the more likely they were to develop type 2 diabetes.

Skip the bacon and hot dogs. While red meat seems to increase the risk of developing diabetes, processed meats such as bacon and hot dogs seem to increase it even more.

Pick up pork chops or a lean pork loin. Pork loin is very lean meat and isn't too expensive. Throw a couple of chops on the grill (dress them up first with a low-calorie garlic–lime juice marinade, or with chili and garlic powders) for a quick dinner—each is just 129 calories, with a healthy 16 grams of protein.

Buy a package of chicken tenderloins to keep in your freezer for quick meals. Each tenderloin weighs about 1½ to 2 ounces, which makes portion control easy for you—two tenderloins are roughly equal to one 3-ounce

Go Lean on Beef

Many cuts of beef are 20 percent leaner than they were 14 years ago—great news if you want to indulge in a steak or beef stew every now and again. The following cuts of beef are listed in order of leanness, and all contain less than 10 grams of total fat, 4.5 grams of saturated fat or less, and fewer than 95 milligrams of cholesterol per serving.

- Eye round roast
- Top round steak
- Mock tender steak
- Bottom round roast
- Top sirloin steak
- Round tip roast

- 95 percent lean ground beef
- Flat half of a brisket
- Shank crosscuts
- Chuck shoulder roast
- Arm pot roast
- Shoulder steak
- Top loin steak (such as strip or New York steak)
- Flank steak
- Rib-eye steak
- Rib steak
- Tri-tip roast
- Tenderloin steak
- T-bone steak

golden rule! Buy Fresh Fish Every Time You Shop

Fatty fish such as mackerel, sardines, herring, salmon, and albacore tuna deliver plenty of protein without saturated fat—and they're excellent sources of omega-3 fatty acids, which slash the risk of heart disease. Equally important, they calm chronic inflammation, common in people with diabetes. (Several large studies found that women with the highest levels of chronic inflammation had a fourfold increased risk for type 2 diabetes.) Scientists aren't sure why, but inflammatory chemicals may interfere with the work of insulin, causing blood sugar to rise. So perhaps it's no coincidence that population studies show that fish lovers have unusually low rates of type 2 diabetes. Your goal: Eating at least two 3.5-ounce servings of fatty fish per week.

serving, which is about the size of a deck of cards. Tenderloins will marinate quickly and can be used in kebabs or tossed into stir-fry dishes.

Choose turkey or chicken breast at the deli counter. Lean slices of meat on whole-wheat bread topped with mustard and baby spinach leaves make a healthy, low-cholesterol lunch—that is, if you select lunch meats that are low in saturated fat. Skip the salamis and bolognas. Good second choices are lean ham and roast beef—just stick to two slices or 1½ ounces of meat in your sandwich.

Go to the freezer section for frozen edamame. These young green soybeans, in or out of their shell, are wonderful as snacks; just steam them and add a little salt. You can also add them to soups and salads. Soy has more protein, by volume, than beef, and virtually none of the saturated fat.

Get your fill of fish from cans or pouches. Salmon is nature's heart medicine, but you don't have to cook up a fillet to get more of it into your diet. Canned salmon is a smart choice not only for convenience but for health; that's because most canned salmon in the United States is wild-caught fish versus farmed fish (and therefore may contain fewer contaminants). An added bonus to eating salmon: Researchers recently found that people who had the highest levels of omega-3 fatty acids in their blood were 53 percent less likely to report feeling mildly or moderately depressed.

Buy seafood to stash in the freezer. Vacuum-packed sole, cod, or salmon fillets, which are flash-frozen, are the next best thing to fresh fish. Keep some in the freezer and you'll always have ingredients for a healthy dinner on hand. You can thaw the fish in the fridge overnight or defrost it under cool running water. Cleaned frozen shrimp is another great buy. Pair it with frozen mixed veggies and you have a stir-fry dinner ready to go.

shop smarter for snacks and sweets

Snacking isn't right for everyone who has diabetes, but for some people, especially those who go more than four or five hours between meals, snacks have a place on the menu. The trick is to choose healthy munchies. Unfortunately, many of the items in the "snack aisle" are filled with cheap ingredients such as high-fructose corn syrup and hydrogenated oil that make good profits for the manufacturers but do little or nothing for you besides upping your consumption of empty calories, dangerous fats, and refined carbohydrates, which wreak havoc on blood sugar and contribute to weight gain. Here's how to select treats that indulge your sweet and salty cravings but won't lead you astray of your dietary goals. (Hint: You'll be venturing outside the snack aisle.)

Head back to the produce department for pre-sliced, pre-washed carrot sticks. Pop them in the front of your fridge or tote them when you're on the go in a zip-close bag for a healthy snack anywhere, anytime. With all their fiber and water, carrots fill your tummy with very few calories.

Say yes to low-fat mozzarella sticks. Snacks low in carbs and moderate in fat are rare birds, but this is one of them. Though the sticks may be a little more expensive than pound-sized blocks of mozzarella ounce for ounce, they're a sound nutritional investment. The 1-ounce servings contain just 70 calories, 4 grams of fat, and less than 1 carbohydrate gram. You'll also know exactly how much cheese you're adding to a whole-wheat pita pizza if you shred one stick, rather than eyeballing a package of grated cheese.

Buy single-serving boxes of raisins. Yes, raisins are higher in sugar than the grapes from which they come. But single-serving boxes will make sure you stick to small portions of this otherwise good-for-you food.

Go nuts (in moderation). Even though nuts are high in calories, studies find that people who eat nuts tend to weigh less. And Harvard researchers found that women who regularly ate about a handful of nuts five times a week were 20 percent less likely to develop type 2 diabetes as those who didn't. The benefits probably come from nuts' blend of protein and good-for-you fats, which make nuts an ideal snack. Just be sure to buy the no-salt versions. Almonds in particular are excellent sources of vitamin E, an antioxidant that may protect against kidney damage and eye and nerve complications.

Choose low-fat, whole-grain crackers. If the cracker you usually eat leaves a ring of oil after you've placed it on a napkin, then you know it's time to switch. Buy a brand that contains at least 3 grams of fiber per serving (about six small crackers). Make sure it doesn't contain any trans fats

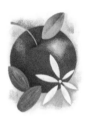

Even though nuts are high in calories, people who eat them tend to weigh less.

golden rule! Check Food Labels for Saturated Fat and Sodium

For people with diabetes, these are the crucially important pieces of data. Why? Diabetes puts you at a higher risk for developing heart disease so no more than 7 percent of your caloric intake should come from saturated fat (for a 2,000-calorie-a-day diet, that's a maximum of 15 grams of fat). And because having diabetes typically means having higher blood pressure, your intake of milligrams of sodium should be equal to or less than the number of calories you eat a day (in other words, no more than 2,000 milligrams of sodium in a 2,000-calorie diet).

(check for the word "hydrogenated" on the ingredient list), which are linked to heart disease.

Buy granola bars, but choose carefully. Some granola bars, with lots of added sugar and little fiber, might as well be candy bars. But if you look hard, you can find a brand that contains no less than 5 grams of fiber and no more than 150 calories per bar. Some high-fiber bars contain as many as 9 grams of appetite-curbing fiber. It also doesn't hurt to see what effect your favorite granola bar has on your blood sugar; just check your blood sugar two hours after eating one. Once you find a good brand, buy a box and stash a few in your handbag or in your glove compartment for quick on-the-go snacks.

Look for 100-calorie snack packs. Snack manufacturers are now offering everything from granola bars and cookies to crackers and potato chips in 100-calorie, snack-pack portions. Though many of these snacks are high in fat and sugar and are therefore best eaten as occasional treats, you can keep your caloric and fat intake in check by occasionally indulging in one of these preportioned bags.

Ignore sales on unhealthy snacks. A "buy one, get one free" sale on potato chips may sound too good to pass up, but it isn't. If you take them home (even if you have the intention of buying them for someone else in the house), you're bound to eat them.

Skip the fat-free cookies. Manufacturers usually just add more sugar to these, and research shows that most people will eat more of them than they would the regular version.

Also skip the sugar-free ice cream. In some cases, manufacturers use sugar alcohols as sweetening agents in sugar-free products, which can cause intestinal gas and diarrhea. People with diabetes may have decreased motility in their gastrointestinal tract as it is, and these foods could make their digestive troubles worse. Also, sugar alcohols contain calories, so though they may be sugar-free, they're not calorie-free and can raise blood sugar. Enjoy a small portion of a reduced-fat ice cream or frozen yogurt instead.

Get your chocolate fix from frozen fudge bars or ice cream sandwiches. Low-fat ice cream sandwiches are lower in carbohydrates, fat, and calories than most chocolate treats. Just avoid ice cream bars covered in a chocolate coating because the coating tends to be made from tropical oils, which are high in saturated fat. At just 88 calories and 1 gram of fat each, Fudgesicles are much better bets than candy bars if you're watching your waistline.

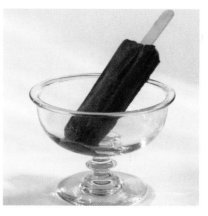

Snack on dark chocolate chips. To satisfy a chocolate craving, dole out five or six of the semisweet chips used to make chocolate-chip cookies. Dark chocolate is extremely rich in antioxidants that protect your heart as well as the rest of your body from cell-damaging free radicals.

Sugar by Any Other Name

Sugar is a simple carbohydrate devoid of any nutritional benefits. And even if an ingredient label doesn't list "sugar," that doesn't mean there isn't any. Manufacturers use more kinds of sugar than you can shake a stick at, and it's worth familiarizing yourself with some of them so you're not fooled into thinking an item is better for you than it is. Look for any of these:

• Amazake

• Brown sugar

• Carob powder

• Corn syrup

• Dextrose

• Evaporated cane juice

• Fructose

• Fruit juice concentrate

• High-fructose corn syrup

• Honey

• Maltose

To get a sense of how much sugar you're really eating, check the nutrition label for "Sugars," listed in grams. Every 4 grams is equivalent to a teaspoon of sugar. Experts suggest we limit our sugar intake to just 12 teaspoons a day from all food sources.

shopping low on the glycemic index

What's the difference between mashed potatoes and spaghetti? The potatoes tend to send blood sugar up high in a hurry, while the pasta causes less of a stir—even if you were to eat the same amount of total carbohydrate in both cases. Scientists have discovered that some types of carbs, once in the body, convert faster to glucose than others do.

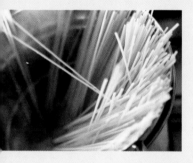

Back in 1981 a nutrition scientist tested a host of foods (all containing 50 grams of carbohydrate) on people, measured the blood sugar reactions, and used them to rate the foods on a scale he called the glycemic index (GI). He discovered that certain starchy foods, such as potatoes and cornflakes, raised blood sugar nearly as much as pure glucose did! These earned high GI scores.

One thing the GI doesn't take into account, though, is how much carbohydrate a serving of a food contains. You'd have to eat a heck of a lot of carrots to get 50 grams of carbs from them. The same goes for most vegetables and fruits. A better measure, then, is the glycemic load (GL), which corrects for this problem.

why are low-GL foods more desirable than high-GL foods?

High-GL foods cause blood glucose levels to rise sharply, prompting the pancreas to secrete insulin to bring it back down. Low-GL foods create a smaller, more sustained rise in blood glucose and don't require as much insulin.

Studies have found that people who eat diets with a high GL have a higher rate of obesity, diabetes, heart disease, and cancer. One study found that men who typically ate foods with a high GL had a 40 percent higher chance of developing diabetes. In the Nurses' Healthy Study, women who ate diets with a high GL had a 37 percent higher chance of getting type 2 diabetes over the six-year span of the study. Yet another study found that swapping just one baked potato per week for a serving of brown rice could reduce a person's odds of developing type 2 diabetes by up to 30 percent.

Of course, eating low-GL can also help if you already have diabetes. In one recent study published in the *American Journal of Clinical Nutrition,* researchers asked volunteers to eat 14 different typical meals (such as bagels and cream cheese with orange juice, for example), then measured the change in their blood glucose levels. They found that the GI of the foods in each meal was about 90 percent accurate in predicting how much the volunteers' glucose levels changed.

can I lose weight eating lower-GL foods?

Maybe. Because they don't trigger blood sugar highs—which are usually followed by lows that cause hunger—low-GL foods keep people full longer. Population studies have shown that people who get most of their carbs from the low end of the GI index tend to weigh less than others who gravitate toward sugary or starchy foods. And one study that compared a low-fat diet with a low-GL diet found that over the course of six to 10 weeks, the people on the low-GL diet reported less hunger, showed better use of insulin, and had less inflammation in their bodies, which translates to a lower risk of artery damage and heart disease.

how do I choose low-GL foods?

First and foremost, choosing low-GL foods means reaching for more fresh, non-starchy fruits and vegetables, nearly all of which fall very low on the GL scale. (Go easier on starchier vegetables including potatoes, parsnips, corn, and peas.) Low-fat dairy foods also tend to be low-GI, along with most protein foods (that makes sense, since it's carbohydrates, not proteins, that raise blood sugar). Choose breakfast cereals with at least 5 grams of fiber per serving, and they will likely be fairly low GL. And opt for whole grains (such as brown rice, barley, bulgur, oatmeal, and coarse whole-wheat bread) over refined grains like white rice and white bread and foods made with white flour, such as most store-bought baked goods. In general, the more finely ground the grain and the less fiber it contains, the faster it will be digested—and the faster blood sugar will rise. That's one reason oatmeal, which isn't ground, has a lower GL than most cold cereals.

which high-GL foods should I avoid?

Nutritionists say "never say never." In other words, no foods are banned completely from a healthy diet. See the chart below for a few foods to cut back on or eat in smaller portion sizes and some comparable choices that don't raise blood sugar as much.

INSTEAD OF ...	TRY
White potatoes or French fries	Sweet potatoes or fries made from sweet potatoes
White rice	Brown or converted rice, quinoa, bulgur, pearled barley, or pasta cooked al dente
White bread	Coarse whole-grain bread, genuine sourdough bread, or dense rye bread
Cornflakes, rice cereal, or instant cream of wheat	Bran cereal, oatmeal, or regular cream of wheat
Corn	Beans and lentils
Chips, pretzels, rice cakes, or jelly beans	Nuts
Sugary beverages or juices	Low-fat or nonfat milk or tomato juice

For more information on the GL of common foods, see pages 266-67.

herbs, spices, and extras

It's often the little things we add to our food that transform a meal from humdrum to high flavor. Herbs and spices are especially valuable, not only because they add taste without fat but also because many have strong antioxidant and anti-inflammatory powers. Condiments like mayonnaise and mustard add tang and texture, but be careful in the condiment aisle or you could end up eating a lot more sugar and salt than you realize.

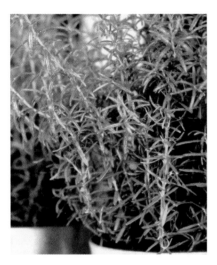

Buy potted herbs and keep them on your kitchen windowsill. If your grocery store sells fresh flowers, chances are they also have potted plants—including culinary herbs. Not only will herbs like oregano, basil, rosemary, and thyme make your kitchen smell nice, they'll be within arm's length whenever you want to flavor your meats and soups without additional fat.

Build up your herb and spice supply with a new selection every week. Do you like your foods hot and spicy or herbaceous? Whatever the case, adding variety to your spice rack can help you add flavor to your food without calories or fat. The next time you're out shopping, bring home ginger, cayenne, turmeric, fresh garlic, minced onion, curry, dried basil, oregano, or rosemary—or something new altogether—and look for clever ways to work them into your meal. For instance, stir half a teaspoon of ground cumin into water before you boil some brown rice, or sprinkle curry rather than salt on your freshly popped popcorn.

Look for fruit- and vegetable-based salsas. If ever there were a low-calorie, versatile condiment, this is it: Salsa is a great topping for baked fish, chicken fajitas, and even baked potatoes. A 2-tablespoon serving of a jarred, tomato-based salsa contains 10 calories and no fat. Think about that the next time you reach for the mayonnaise, which packs 114 calories and 10 grams of fat in 2 tablespoons.

Seek out flaxseeds. You can easily add more fiber to any meal or snack by adding 1 or 2 teaspoons of ground flaxseeds. An easy way to remember their benefits is "1-1-1": Each teaspoon of flaxseed has 1 gram of fat, 1 gram of fiber, and 1 gram of protein (and only 17 calories). Purchase ground seeds or grind your own in a clean coffee grinder. Add them to smoothies, salads, casseroles, and baked goods batter. Just make sure to store them in the refrigerator after opening. A word of warning: Eat too many flaxseeds and you'll quickly discover their laxative effect.

Read condiment labels for calories and sodium. If a tablespoon of the condiment is less than 25 calories, you probably don't need to bother counting those carbs if you're counting carbs (see page 52). But with some condiments, such as mayonnaise or mustards mixed with oils, the calories can add up fast, so buy something else, or plan to use it in very small portions. Sodium is the other hidden hazard. A tablespoon of ketchup can contain 190 milligrams of sodium. Some salad dressings are even bigger offenders. Choose low-sodium versions whenever possible (or make your own salad dressing). Remember that a food should have no more milligrams of sodium than it has calories.

Choose mustard over ketchup. Most mustards contain no added sugar, and they're much lower in sodium than ketchup is.

Substitute low-fat yogurt for mayonnaise. When you do this, it's best to drain a bit of the liquid from the yogurt. Line a sieve with a large coffee filter or two layers of white paper towels (avoid printed ones). Place the sieve over a large bowl. Place 1 cup of yogurt in the filter. Refrigerate for about 3 hours. This will yield ½ cup "yogurt cheese."

Grab a few heads of garlic. It may just be one of the perfect herbs for people with diabetes. Scientific studies show that garlic may increase insulin secretion, which lowers blood sugar; garlic also modestly lowers "bad" cholesterol and "thins" the blood to help prevent dangerous clots. And it's packed with antioxidants, which help stave off diabetes-related complications. As flavorful and beneficial as garlic is, it should be one of the first items you toss into your grocery basket. It's delicious roasted and used as a spread on meat or bread. Minced garlic, too, jazzes up salad dressings, sautéed vegetables, meat marinades, and more.

Stock up on lemon pepper. It's a wonderful way to add flavor, not sodium, to vegetables, meats, and starches.

Switch to kosher salt. Because it's coarser, there's less of it by volume compared to regular table salt. In fact, there's nearly half the sodium in 1 tablespoon of kosher salt than in table salt.

Try blackened seasoning. These spice mixes lend serious kick to fish, chicken, or shrimp without fat or calories. They usually contain cayenne pepper, black pepper, garlic and onion powder, and possibly paprika, celery or fennel seeds, and other ingredients. If you like spicy food that's not too hot, there's no better way to quickly add a lot flavor. Also try other dry rubs, such as cracked pepper rubs. Go for the better brands; they often rely less on salt for their taste.

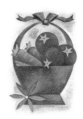

Garlic may increase insulin secretion, which lowers blood sugar.

navigate the beverage aisles

If you have diabetes, figuring out what to drink can be tricky. Soft drinks (other than diet varieties) contain far too much sugar and too many calories, and even 100 percent fruit juice should be rationed because it's higher in sugar than real fruit and contains none of the fiber. Read on for some smart suggestions.

Buy pomegranate juice and dilute it. This juice is particularly high in antioxidants, but like other fruit juices, it's too high in calories. Plan to dilute it with water (at least 50 percent water) and ice.

Stock up on tea. If you're limiting your intake of soda and other sweetened drinks, and you don't always care for plain water, what can you drink? Tea! It's rich in antioxidants that help protect your arteries and stave off complications of diabetes. For extra convenience when you want to brew your own tea, try cold-brew tea bags—just one bag turns a glass of ice water into a calorie-free tea. Of course you can also find many varieties of ready-to-drink unsweetened ice tea, including green teas. Just avoid sweetened iced teas.

Look for calorie-free flavored waters that aren't carbonated. Unlike seltzers and club sodas, these aren't high in sodium.

Try tomato juice. It's a good way to sneak a vegetable serving into your day, and it has less of an effect on blood sugar than fruit juices do. That said, tomato juice tends to be awfully high in sodium, so look for a low-sodium variety or add water to regular tomato juice to dilute it.

If you buy soft drinks, make sure they're diet. Soda is filled with calories empty on nutrition. Drinking it raises the risk of both diabetes and obesity. If you must drink it, make it diet and spare yourself the calories.

chapter two

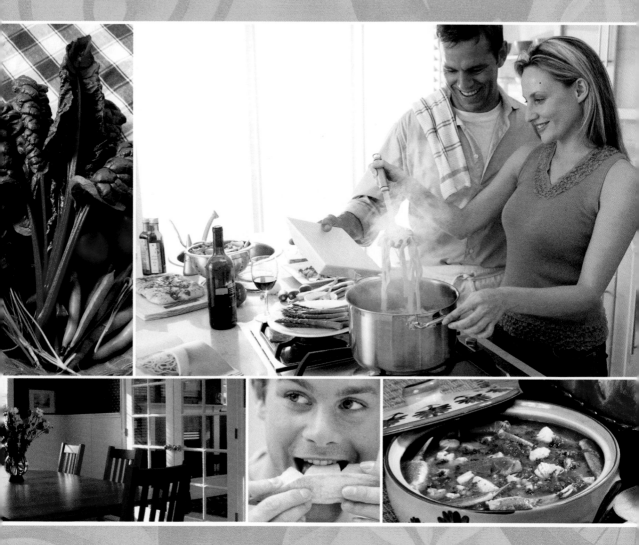

in your kitchen

Consider your kitchen ground zero for managing your diabetes.
After all, in many ways this is a disease that begins—
and ends—with food. In this chapter we'll reveal our best
secrets for doing what it takes to beat diabetes as
the *chef de cuisine* of your own home.

stock and streamline your cooking space

If success at any goal starts with a ready mind, success at beating diabetes starts with a ready kitchen. It's a simple law of human behavior: The easier and more convenient it is to do something, the more likely you are to do it. Your goal, then, is to set up a kitchen that lets you whip up healthy meals in a hurry and reach first for diabetes-friendly snacks and beverages. Here's how to stack the "decks" of your kitchen in your favor.

Many herbs and spices have powers that can help you control diabetes.

Keep the kitchen clean. Make a rule and share it with every member of the family: Dirty dishes are never to be left in the sink, and the counters and table are to remain clean. You'll be far more motivated to cook healthy meals if you don't have to clean the kitchen first.

Place an enticing pitcher of water in the fridge. Take your prettiest pitcher, fill it with ice, water, and lemon wedges, and place it front and center in the fridge. Whenever you open the refrigerator out of boredom, pour yourself a glass of water. Researchers in Germany studied people's metabolism after they drank about 17 ounces of water. Within 10 minutes of taking the drink, they burned 30 percent more calories than before they drank the water, and the boost in their metabolism lasted for 30 to 40 minutes. Another bonus: Water flushes impurities from your body, important for people with diabetes, who have a high risk of developing kidney disease. Drinking plenty of fluids also guards against water retention, a common problem when kidneys aren't functioning at their optimum capacity.

Keep a fruit bowl or plate on the counter. Make fruits such as apples, pears, peaches, and kiwis the first foods you see when you enter the house ravenous at the end of the day or swing by the kitchen for a snack. A flatter bowl is better than a deep one because most fruits keep best unstacked.

Stock the spice rack. Spices will help you flavor meals without adding fat or calories. Keep dry rubs for meats, Italian seasoning, lemon-herb seasoning, and other favorites in a spice rack on your kitchen counter or tucked in your pantry door for easy access. Some spices—including ginger, cayenne, turmeric, fresh garlic, minced onion, curry, basil, oregano, and rosemary—have anti-inflammatory and antioxidant powers, both of which help with diabetes. Keep these handy to flavor meats and vegetables.

Save a special place for cinnamon sticks. Of all of the spices you have on hand, cinnamon should be one that you reach for every day. A study at the Beltsville Human Nutrition Research Center in Maryland found that consuming as little as half a teaspoon of cinnamon in capsule form can lower fasting blood glucose levels up to 30 percent. Added bonus: The same study showed cinnamon also lowered "bad" cholesterol by up to 27 percent and total cholesterol by as much as 26 percent. Note that the type of cinnamon used in the study was a Chinese cinnamon called *Cinnamomum cassia*.

Keep a small bottle of olive oil on the counter. Olive oil's rich in healthy monounsaturated fats, which, unlike the saturated fat in butter, won't increase your insulin resistance (which raises blood sugar) and will protect your heart from heart disease. Because heat and light can turn olive oil rancid over time, keep a larger bottle in the fridge to refill your countertop bottle. Olive oil will become cloudy in the fridge, but bringing it to room temperature will restore its clarity.

Be sure to use extra-virgin olive oil. Because extra-virgin olive oil comes from the first pressing of olives and contains no refined oils, it has high levels of phenols, antioxidants that help prevent high cholesterol, high blood pressure, and heart disease, as well as complications of diabetes, such as nerve problems.

Stock your fridge with trans fat-free margarine. Trans fats, which are made when vegetable oils are hydrogenated and turned into solid fats, are considered deadly by many experts because they significantly increase the risk of heart disease. If you have high cholesterol, opt instead for a spread that contains plant sterols or stanols. They actually block the amount of cholesterol absorbed by the small intestines.

Toss out your corn oil. Corn oil doesn't stand up to olive oil when you compare their health benefits. Olive oil contains 72 percent monounsaturated fats, while corn oil contains only 24 percent, so olive oil does a better job of lowering cholesterol. Even more important, olive oil fights inflammation in the body, which is linked to many diseases including diabetes and heart disease, whereas corn oil is thought by many health experts to promote inflammation. When olive oil won't do in a recipe, such as in baking, use canola oil. It has a milder taste than olive oil but also contains an impressive amount of heart-healthy monounsaturated fat.

make the change!

The habit: Switching to olive oil.

The result: Lower blood pressure and cholesterol.

The proof: In a study of men who don't normally consume olive oil, adding about 2 tablespoons a day to their diets over three weeks lowered their systolic blood pressure (the first number in a blood pressure reading) by 3 percent. This is especially important for people with type 2 diabetes because the disease puts you at higher risk of developing hypertension. In a separate study, adding 2 tablespoons of olive oil a day for six weeks led to a 12 percent drop in total cholesterol and a 16 percent drop in LDL ("bad" cholesterol). Olive oil also raises HDL, or "good" cholesterol. Another healthy option is canola oil, also rich in monounsaturated fat and usually cheaper. Remember that 2 tablespoons of oil contains approximately 270 calories, so you'll need to use the oil in place of, not in addition to, other fats.

Keep several kinds of vinegar on hand, such as cider, white, rice, balsamic, and red and white wine vinegars. They'll come in handy for making quick salad dressings and marinades for meat or vegetables. And they bring an extra bonus: Some early research suggests that adding acids to meals (think vinegar as well as lemon juice) blunts the effect of the meal on your blood sugar. Try balsamic vinegar on top of sliced strawberries for an unexpected taste sensation.

Plant healthy snacks within sight. You know you shouldn't be eating cookies, so why did you pop one into your mouth the second you walked

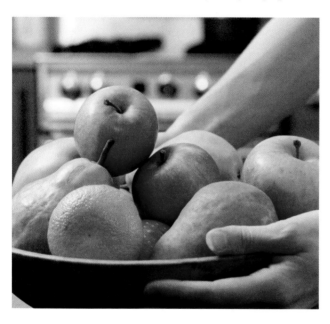

into the kitchen? Maybe because the open package was sitting in the front of your cabinet, taunting you. Banish the cookies to the back of a high shelf or even the freezer. Put in their place some almonds, walnuts, and peanuts. Also stash some low-fat yogurt in the front of the fridge, and keep some cut-up carrot sticks or a bowl of cherry tomatoes or sugar snap peas there, too.

Better yet, banish junk food from the kitchen. If your family insists on having bags of sugary, salty, fatty snacks around the house, tell them to store the snacks where you won't find them. Hiding places outside of the kitchen are best. Tell your spouse to stash his or her chips in the garage or the trunk of the car.

Stock some meal replacement drinks made for people with diabetes. You'll read soon how important it is to eat breakfast every day. "Real" food is always preferable to meal replacement drinks, but for those mornings when you really don't have time even for a bowl of cereal, keep some canned drinks or shakes ready to grab and go. Beverages made by Glucerna and Choice DM are designed for people with diabetes. They contain slow-digesting carbs, and often some fiber, so they don't cause blood sugar to rise quite as high or as fast as other similar drinks.

Keep at least one emergency meal in the freezer. Forgot to buy chicken for Tuesday night's chicken marsala? No sweat. Individual servings of vegetable lasagna await in the freezer. Just heat and serve. When you run

whip it together! Fix-It-and-Forget-It Freezer Casserole

One bowl, one oven, and one freezer. Could cooking be any simpler? Prepare this fiber-rich casserole when you have some extra time. On days you can't spare a minute to cook, pop it out of the freezer and into the oven.

2 cups cooked **brown rice**

1 package (10 ounces) **frozen corn**, thawed

1 cup diced **white meat turkey**

⅓ cup diced **onion**

4 ounces shredded reduced-fat **cheddar cheese**

1 cup fat-free **milk**

½ teaspoon **chili powder**

Salt and **pepper** to taste

Combine all ingredients in a large bowl. Pour into a nonstick 2-quart casserole dish. Bake at 350°F for 40 to 45 minutes. Remove from the oven, let cool slightly, cover, and wrap in heavy-duty foil. Place in the freezer for up to 2 months. When ready to serve, remove to the refrigerator and thaw overnight. Bake at 325°F for 25 minutes until heated through.

out of back-ups, make a double batch of your next meal and freeze the extra. Casseroles, soups, and cooked meat can be frozen for up to three months. Use plastic bags and wrap made specifically for the freezer or store in airtight freezer containers.

Buy a vegetable steamer. It's the healthiest way to cook vegetables because nutrients aren't lost in the water. Choose a metal steamer basket (fill it with veggies, place over a saucepan of rapidly simmering water, cover, and cook for 5 to 10 minutes) or a microwave steamer (add a small amount of water to the bottom of the container, add veggies to the basket, and cook for two to five minutes).

Keep an electric flaxseed, spice, or coffee grinder on the counter. Any of them will grind whole flaxseeds and make it convenient for you to add these important sources of fiber and omega-3 fatty acids to your cereal, salad, yogurt, and baked good batter. Although you can buy flaxseed that has already been ground, it won't have as much flavor as freshly ground, and it will spoil faster.

plan your meals

You wouldn't start a vacation without an idea of where you're going to go, and neither should you start your day or week without an idea of what you're going to eat. We're not saying you have to plan every bite, but with so many unhealthy choices all-too-readily available (you probably pass a few fast-food joints whenever you drive your car and stare down dough-nuts when you buy your morning paper), having a plan, writing it down, and sticking to it is the smart approach.

Set aside time on Sunday to plan your menu for the next seven days. Look through cookbooks, recipe cards, or the latest issue of a healthy cooking magazine, and pick out seven healthy dinners with reasonable calorie totals, usually no more than about 500 calories per serving. Remember to include a lean protein source (such as chicken breast, fish, or beans), plenty of vegetables, and a whole-grain source of fiber. Breakfasts and lunches can be a little more spontaneous, but it's still a good to have a general idea of what you'll be eating (oatmeal or cereal with fruit in the mornings, salads and soups for lunch, etc.) so you're not caught off guard and unprepared.

Write out a grocery list based on your week's menu. Take it to the store and don't buy anything that's not on the list (unless of course you forgot to write down basics like milk and toilet paper). Now even if your week

Secrets from a Chef with Diabetes

What does a chef do when he learns he has diabetes? Franklin Becker, chef of the 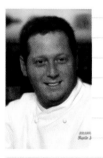 Brasserie restaurant in New York City and author of *The Diabetic Chef*, put his cooking skills to the test. A lover of double plates of pasta and multiple slices of pizza, Becker decided to overhaul his eating habits, adding serious amounts of vegetables and cutting back on carbs. Soon his body began adapting. He felt fuller on smaller portions, and he felt more energized.

Today, he has good control over his blood sugar. Here, a few of Becker's simple recipes.

Pizza, Downsized

Brush a flour tortilla with olive oil and layer slices of tomatoes, thinly sliced or grated part-skim mozzarella cheese, and fresh basil. Heat in the oven until the cheese melts.

Steamy, Flavorful Vegetables

Add a bit of water to a saucepan with a teaspoon of olive oil, sea salt, and any kind of vegetable, such as sugar snap peas, broccoli, or cauliflower. Cook the water and oil down

turns busy and exhausting, you won't have to shop or wonder what you should make for dinner. A healthy meal is already planned and ready to cook!

Buy a set of magnetic clips and use them to hang your recipes for the week on the fridge. It will be one more reminder that you have a healthy meal planned before you have a chance to open the drawer for a take-out menu.

Put fish on the menu twice a week. Eating up to two servings of fish—especially fatty fish like salmon, tuna, or mackerel—will supply enough omega-3 fatty acids to cut your risk of dying of a heart attack by 30 percent. One way omega-3 fatty acids help lower heart attack risk is by fighting inflammation in the arteries and elsewhere. Another upside to "fin food": If you're eating fish, that means you're not eating a fatty steak or an oversize plate of macaroni and cheese, both diabetes disasters.

Enjoy a Greek "picnic" on Thursdays. Start with a homemade Greek salad that includes lettuce, chopped juicy tomatoes, cubed cucumbers, a handful of chickpeas, 3 ounces of grilled chicken per person, and an ounce of low-fat feta cheese per person. Drizzle with olive oil and vinegar and add pickled pepperoncini hot peppers, if you like them. As a side dish, serve tzatziki, made with 2 cups of strained Greek yogurt, several cloves of diced

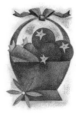

Eating fatty fish can cut your risk of dying of a heart attack.

until it thickens and forms a bit of a sauce. Finish it off with chopped fresh parsley, chives, and tarragon.

Orange and Arugula Salad

Toss arugula leaves with orange segments, freshly squeezed lemon, and a drizzle of olive oil. "The lemon cuts through the peppery taste of the arugula, and it's a delicious salad with nothing more added to it," Becker says.

A Smooth, Filling Vegetable Soup

Fill a saucepan with water, add a head of chopped cauliflower, a couple of chopped leeks, and a clove of garlic. Cover the pan and boil the water until the cauliflower is tender. Cool slightly and transfer the soup to a blender. Add some salt, a touch of clarified butter, and a pinch of curry powder. Puree and serve.

A No-Bread Sandwich

Sauté boneless chicken breast with ginger, garlic, scallions, and soy sauce. Then wrap it in a large lettuce leaf. "Sprinkle on some toasted cashews or peanuts, and it's even better," Becker says.

garlic, ½ cup of peeled, diced, or shredded cucumber, 1 tablespoon of olive oil, 2 teaspoons of lemon juice, and chopped mint to taste. Put out warmed whole-grain flat bread, and top it off with a glass of red wine or unsweetened iced tea. Eating Mediterranean-style is good for your heart and may improve insulin resistance.

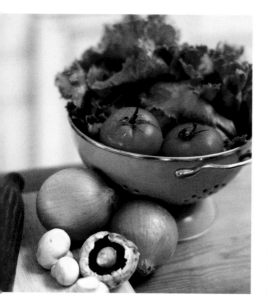

Toss a big salad on Sunday. Lettuce and most crisp vegetables will remain fresh for several days in the refrigerator, so making a big salad on Sunday should get you through until Wednesday or Thursday. Mix diced carrots, celery, green beans, fresh broccoli, and cauliflower with your favorite greens and store in an airtight container. Add anything that contains moisture, such as tomatoes, cucumbers, olives, low-fat cheese, chicken, tuna, or turkey, just before serving.

Prep for tomorrow the night before. Take 20 minutes from your evening TV viewing to do some prep work that will make the next day go smoothly. Hard-boil eggs for breakfast and put them in the fridge, set the breakfast table, cut up fruit for your cereal, and set the coffee machine. Planning a berry crisp for dinner Friday night? On Thursday, measure and pour the flour, oatmeal, cinnamon, and other spices into a plastic bag and seal. The next day you'll simply have to throw it together with the berries and bake.

Buy a dry-erase board from an office supply store and use it to track your servings of fiber-rich foods. Getting more fiber into your diet is one of the best ways to shrink your waistline and lower your blood sugar, but it's probably not top-of-mind when you're looking for something to eat. The answer? Every day, write down every fiber-rich food that passes your lips: Your morning bowl of oatmeal (give yourself an extra fiber food for adding fruit or flaxseeds on top), your sandwich on two pieces of whole-grain bread (that counts as two) your afternoon apple, your sides of brown rice and steamed spinach at dinner. Aim for at least eight. The visual reminder will spur you to eat more servings as the day progresses if you see you're falling short. Need one last serving after dinner? Snack on air-popped popcorn in the evening.

make breakfast count

Breakfast sounds like the easiest meal of the day, and in fact it is. It's also your best chance to increase the fiber in your diet, since the menu includes so many high-fiber choices like oatmeal and whole-grain cereal. And it's an excellent opportunity to get at least one serving of fruit (what's better on top of that oatmeal or cereal?) and one serving of dairy (what else would you pour into your cereal but milk?). A bonus to eating breakfast: It kick-starts your metabolism again after a night of fasting.

Eat breakfast at home. You can't (and shouldn't) avoid restaurants altogether, but there's one meal you should almost always eat at home: breakfast. Look at the alternatives: Diner-style breakfasts can include 1,000 calories or more with astronomical amounts of carbohydrates and fat. A healthy-sounding whole-wheat bagel with light cream cheese from a bagel shop may contain up to 67 grams of carbs, 450 calories, and 9 grams of fat. A sausage muffin may pack 29 grams of carbs, 370 calories, and 22 grams of fat. Compare those to a bowl of oatmeal (half a cup) with a half cup of fat-free milk, which contains a mere 12 grams of carbs, 195 calories, and 3 grams of fat.

Always top your cereal with fruit. We assume you're already starting out with a cereal that contains at least 5 grams of fiber per serving. (Studies have found that people who regularly eat whole-grain cereal gain less weight than people who don't.) Make it even more diabetes-friendly by adding half a cup (one serving) of fresh fruit, such as strawberries or blueberries.

Sprinkle 1 or 2 tablespoons of ground flaxseed on hot and cold cereal and yogurt. Rich in protein and fiber, these tiny seeds are a godsend to your blood sugar as well as your heart. They also contain fatty acids that the body uses to make the same type of omega-3 fatty acids you get from fish. Like fish, the seeds lower cholesterol and help guard against inflammation. Plus their slightly nutty taste is delicious! Store whole seeds in the fridge, and grind the amount you need with a spice or coffee grinder.

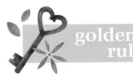
golden rule!   ## Always Eat Breakfast

Even if your blood sugar is high in the morning, don't skip breakfast. Research shows that forgoing a morning meal increases the risk for obesity and insulin resistance. And studies confirm that breakfast eaters are better able to resist fatty and high-calorie foods later in the day. Aim to eat your breakfast at the same time every day, since keeping your blood sugar levels even throughout the day means eating consistently from day to day.

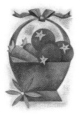

Vitamin D, which is added to fortified milk, helps your body use insulin.

Have oatmeal several days a week, especially in winter. Oatmeal's one of the best breakfasts you can eat if you have diabetes. It contains 4 grams of fiber per cup, which will help keep blood sugar levels steady. And studies have shown that eating a cup of oatmeal five or six times a week can lower the risk of developing type 2 diabetes by 39 percent. Oatmeal also may help you eat less later in the day. One study found that people who ate oatmeal in the morning ate 30 percent fewer calories at lunch compared with people who ate sugared, flaked cereal for breakfast.

Cook a large batch of steel-cut oatmeal on Sunday mornings. Enjoy one serving, and then refrigerate the rest. On weekday mornings, simply reheat in the microwave. Add raisins and cinnamon if you like. This will save loads of time because steel-cut oatmeal takes as long as 50 minutes to cook.

Make your own flavored oatmeal. Instead of buying packets of flavored oatmeal, which usually contain added sugar and salt and use more-processed oats, make your own oatmeal with few flavor boosters—and few diabetes busters! Start with old-fashioned or steel-cut oats and add chopped apples or peaches for sweetness (and fiber) and a generous sprinkling of blood-sugar-lowering cinnamon.

Have nonfat milk or yogurt with breakfast. When researchers studied 10,000 women, they found that the more calcium and vitamin D (which is added to fortified milk) the women consumed, the less likely they were to have metabolic syndrome, a cluster of symptoms that increases the risk of diabetes and heart disease. Vitamin D also helps the body use insulin, and consuming more calcium is associated with lower cholesterol levels. Drinking milk and eating dairy products help people lose weight, too.

Choose plain, nonfat yogurt over fruit yogurt. You can save 11 grams of carbohydrates this way. And don't be fooled into thinking that vanilla yogurt has the same calories as plain; a cup of low-fat plain yogurt contains about 50 calories less than a cup of low-fat vanilla.

Have an orange instead of orange juice. Juice is a source of concentrated carbs and lacks the fiber of the whole fruit. And the fruit will make you feel more satisfied and full.

When you drink juice, use a real juice glass. It's just 4 ounces. Fill it with orange juice, which contains 12 grams of carbs, instead of grape juice, which contains 16 grams of carbs.

Doctor your tea or coffee with cinnamon. One way to get more blood-sugar-lowering cinnamon is to add a cinnamon stick to your tea, or make a cinnamon tea by stirring a cinnamon stick in a cup of hot water. Or add half a teaspoon powdered cinnamon to ground coffee before starting the pot.

reinvent your lunch

You plan your dinners (hopefully), but lunch is all too often an after-thought. No problem! Like breakfast, lunch is a pretty simple meal to prepare, and if you follow a few pearls of wisdom, it will take you a long way toward getting the foods that will help you control your diabetes—and keep you full at least until it's time for a small, midday snack. Your goal: Include plenty of fiber (from salads, bean soups, or whole-grain sandwich bread), vegetables, and at least one source of lean protein (such as tuna or grilled chicken).

Swap the full-fat cheese slices in your sandwich for avocado slices. Yes, dairy foods are especially important if you have diabetes, but cheese has a shortcoming: It's loaded with saturated fat, which makes blood sugar control more difficult by making insulin sensitivity worse. Avocados, on the other hand, are high in monounsaturated fats, which help you control your blood sugar and protect your heart. Their creamy richness mimics that of cheese. You don't need to eliminate cheese from your diet completely, just favor cheeses that taste good in lower-fat forms, such as part-skim mozzarella.

Fatten up sandwiches with vegetables. There's nothing wrong with two slices of lean lunch meat such as roast turkey or lean ham in your sandwich—in fact, these are great sources of protein—but most store-bought sandwiches contain at least twice that much meat, not to mention all that mayonnaise and cheese. Don't let your sandwich be a glorification of saturated fat! Make it at home (or custom-order it at the deli), keep the meat lean (no salami or pepperoni!) and modest, and pile on the veggies. Don't stop with lettuce and tomato. Other great sandwich inserts are cucumbers, onions, bean sprouts, and roasted red or yellow peppers.

Add a smear of hummus. It's another fantastic sandwich filler and a great opportunity to eat your beans. Spread it onto a veggie or chicken sandwich for extra protein and fiber. To make your own hummus, pour a can of garbanzo beans into your blender or food processor and add a tablespoon of olive oil and two cloves of chopped garlic. Add lemon juice to taste. Blend and enjoy. Traditionally, hummus is made with tahini, a paste made from ground sesame seeds, but it's not necessary (and it adds a lot of fat). Keep your portion size to 2 or 3 tablespoons' worth.

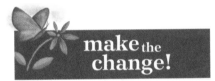

make the change!

The habit: Eating at least three daily servings of whole grains.

The results: Lower blood sugar and a lower risk of metabolic syndrome and heart disease.

The proof: In one study of more than 750 men and women over age 60, those who ate about three servings of whole grains a day were 54 percent less likely to have metabolic syndrome, had lower fasting blood sugar levels and less body fat, and suffered 52 percent fewer fatal heart attacks than people who ate less than one serving a day. A serving of whole grain is one slice of whole-grain bread, a half cup of whole-wheat pasta, or a half cup of brown rice, bulgur, barley, or other whole grain.

Use water-packed tuna on salads and in sandwiches. Albacore tuna contains all-important healthy omega-3 fatty acids, which fight inflammation and help prevent disease. But make sure you buy the tuna packed in water, not oil. Three ounces of water-packed tuna contain less than a gram of fat and 99 calories; the same amount of oil-packed tuna contains 7 grams of fat and 168 calories.

Dress your sandwich with mustard, not mayo. Mustard has none of the fat that mayo has. A tablespoon of yellow mustard has about 11 calories compared to 100 calories in the same amount of mayo.

Add fruit to greens. Sneak in a serving of fruit with your salad! Toss slices of oranges, grapefruit, nectarines, or apples, or strawberries or blueberries, to salads dressed with a vinaigrette and, for a protein boost, sprinkle with roasted walnuts or almonds.

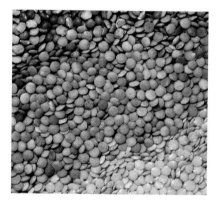

Load up on lentils. Among legumes, lentils are some of the richest in protein. If you're not already eating them, crank open a can of lentil soup and enjoy a small bowl with your salad or sandwich. Or pair just about any lunch or dinner with a lentil salad. Lentils cook quickly and you don't need to soak them first. Their soluble fiber content allows them to digest slowly, so they have a blunting effect on your blood sugar.

Have a salad topped with rinsed canned beans. A large salad at lunch can knock off several vegetable servings in one fell swoop, but don't forget to add protein to keep you full longer. Beans add the perfect heft—both protein and fiber—to your lunch. Try kidney beans, chickpeas, or black beans (especially good if you're adding avocado to your salad).

Buy a sandwich grill. Sometimes a hot sandwich is more satisfying than a cold one, even if it contains the same number of calories. These grills, also called panini grills or sandwich presses, toast sandwiches nicely and melt any cheese you've added. Try cooked chicken breast with tomato and spinach (add a little part-skim mozzarella if you like) or lean, low-salt ham and low-fat Brie. Buy a grill with removable nonstick grill plates to make cleanup easy.

make dinner more diabetes friendly

If your diet is the foundation for beating diabetes, your dinners are the cornerstone. Here's where most of us go overboard on calories, carbs, and fat. That doesn't relegate you to rabbit food. Your dinners can be flavorful and satisfying without wreaking havoc with your blood sugar. Here are some ways to do it.

Make a deal with your spouse. The idea of preparing a meal, washing the dishes, and cleaning the kitchen can be a deal-breaker when it comes to cooking a healthy meal. But before you forgo your eating plan and decide to have frozen pizza, tell your spouse that you'll cook if he'll clean. You'll both benefit from the home-cooked meal, and you'll be able to put up your feet afterward.

Cook once, eat twice. Make double and you'll have dinner for tomorrow. Or pack it up and freeze for a day when you don't have time to cook.

Make a pot of tea before you start cooking. Cooks nibble. It's unconscious, and it's incessant. You can consume several hundred calories in no time tasting the soup, sampling the roast, stealing a little cheese, noshing while you wait for the water to boil. Controlling this is critical for people who cook regularly—and this should include you! Steep a pot of tea before you even begin and turn to your mug instead of your food while you cook.

Start with a simple salad. You'll eat less of the main meal and take in more vegetables to boot. Dress it with a splash of vinegar or lemon juice or an olive oil vinaigrette—not a creamy dressing.

Use your veggie of the week. In the grocery shopping chapter we suggested you designate a vegetable of the week. Don't let it rot in your

whip it together! Garlicky Green Beans

With this "master" recipe, you can take all kinds of vegetables and infuse them with the heady aroma of garlic and onions. Try broccoli, cauliflower, sliced asparagus, or sliced bell peppers in place of the green beans.

Steam 1 pound trimmed **green beans** for 5 minutes over boiling water. Remove from the heat and plunge the green beans in a bowl of ice water to stop the cooking. Drain again and set aside. In a medium skillet, heat 2 teaspoons **olive oil**. Add 1 small diced **onion** and 3 finely minced **garlic** cloves and sauté 3 minutes. Add in 1 can (15 ounces) drained diced **tomatoes** and the reserved green beans. Cook for 2 minutes.

fridge! If it's bok choy, add a handful to soup (homemade or canned) on Monday; sauté it with garlic and 1 teaspoon olive oil on Tuesday; chop it small and add to spaghetti sauce on Wednesday; add it to a stir-fry on Thursday; and try it on pizza (with whole-wheat crust) on Friday. If you juice, add both the stalk and the leaves to your juicer and drink to its vitamin C and fiber content.

Go vegetarian at least once a week. You'll get much more fiber and far less saturated fat. Instead of meat lasagna, have vegetable lasagna using eggplant or a mix of veggies such as broccoli, carrots, bell peppers, mushrooms, and zucchini. Likewise, vegetable chili is a perfectly tasty alternative to meat chili.

Replace a pat with a spray. Take food that's typically fried in butter or oil, such as Italian zucchini patties, and brown them on the stove top with a little cooking spray, suggests Mary Jean Christian, RD, CDE, diabetes education program coordinator at the Joslin Diabetes Center at the University of California, Irvine. She uses cooking spray to brown her grandmother-in-law's zucchini patties instead of using the loads of oil her husband's family traditionally uses for the recipe. The result? Her in-laws say her zucchini patties taste the closest to their grandmother's!

Savor the crunch of oven-baked chicken and fries. Add fried chicken and French fries back into your diet without overloading on saturated fat. Dip strips of boneless, skinless chicken into a little flour, coat in egg beaters, yogurt, or fat-free milk, and cover with plain breadcrumbs mixed with herbs. Then bake in the oven at 350°F for 20 to 30 minutes. The chicken will have a crispy coating that satisfies your yen for fried chicken. For the French fries, cut white or sweet potatoes into strips, soak in water for 20 minutes, and spread them on a baking sheet. Drizzle with olive oil, sprinkle with salt and pepper, and bake for 40 minutes at 350°F, stirring halfway through.

golden rule! Fill Half Your Plate with Vegetables

If you want to see a nice full plate in front of you, fill half of it with non-starchy veggies (that means no potatoes or corn). Split the other half between a protein, such as roasted chicken, and a starch, such as a half cup of brown rice. That will give you two servings of vegetables—and automatically make sure you don't overdo it on carbs. Add a side salad and now you have three vegetable servings in your meal.

whip it together! | Tropical Fruit Salsa

This hot and sweet salsa, loaded with vitamin C, adds an extra-special finish to broiled chicken or fish.

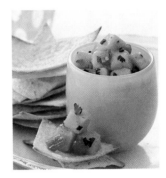

⅔ cup fresh chopped **pineapple** or **mango**

1 **kiwi**, peeled and diced

1 small **orange**, peeled and diced

1 teaspoon seeded and minced **jalapeño pepper**

1 tablespoon minced **red onion**

1 tablespoon minced **red bell pepper**

1 tablespoon fresh **lime juice**

1 teaspoon **sugar** or **sugar substitute**

Combine all the ingredients in a bowl. Cover and refrigerate 1 hour. Serve alongside or on top of broiled chicken or fish. For extra flavor, add 1 tablespoon of chopped fresh cilantro, mint, or parsley.

When beef is on the menu, choose lean cuts. These include filet mignon, flank steak, and round and loin cuts. Remember that a serving of meat is no more than 3 ounces cooked, 4 ounces raw. Steer clear of ribs, prime rib, skirt steak, and brisket.

Put your meals "to bed"—on a bed of greens. Chefs everywhere are serving this or that dish on a bed of greens. You can too! Simply steam some spinach, kale, or Swiss chard on the stove, then put it on your plate and place your fish or chicken on top. When you tire of dark leafy greens, get creative and make your "bed" of steamed snow peas, sugar snap peas, and pea sprouts.

Top fish or chicken with fruit salsa. It's an exciting way to sneak in a serving of fruit and give simple dishes flavor without fat. And what a difference it makes to a piece of fish or a grilled or roasted chicken breast. Make a fruity salsa by combining chunks of pineapple, mango, or papaya with chopped onions, ginger, garlic, mint, cilantro, and hot pepper flakes. Let it sit for 30 minutes at room temperature or up to 4 hours in the fridge.

Make a fruit glaze to drizzle over fish. Try this simple recipe from Deborah Carabet, chef and nutritionist in Los Angeles, California: To a saucepan add a quarter cup of orange juice or water, a half cup of mango fruit spread

(continued on page 54)

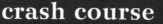
carbohydrate counting

Because carbohydrates raise blood sugar, managing your carbs is key to managing your diabetes. One way to do it is through carbohydrate counting. Knowing how many carbs you can have throughout the day—and following those guidelines consistently every day—will set your blood sugar levels on an even keel, make you feel more energized, and help you avoid complications of diabetes.

Most of the foods you eat—from milk and fruit to breads and grains—contain carbohydrates. There's no way to avoid them, and you wouldn't want to. Carbs serve as the main fuel source for your body. The trick is to avoid eating too many carbs in one day or at one sitting.

When you eat carbs, your body breaks the food down into glucose, which enters the bloodstream. That triggers your pancreas to release the hormone insulin, which helps move the glucose into your cells for energy. The more carbohydrates you eat, the more insulin your body needs to help convert the food to energy.

When you have diabetes, your pancreas doesn't produce enough insulin or your body can't use the insulin to move the glucose into the cells. Starved cells make you feel tired and sluggish. And chronically high blood sugar levels boost the production of free radicals and lower your immunity, on top of other negative effects.

The key, then, is to gain better control over your blood sugar levels by learning just how many carbohydrates you should eat throughout the day. Here's what to do.

1| determine your activity level factor

This is based on your gender and your level of physical activity. The more active you are, the more calories—and carbs—you can eat. If you're a couch potato, rate yourself "sedentary." If you

exercise occasionally, rate yourself "lightly active." If you exercise regularly, you're "active." If you exercise strenuously almost every day, you're "very active."

Activity Level	Female	Male
sedentary	12	13
lightly active	14	15
active	16	17
very active	19	19

2| calculate your daily calorie needs

Multiply your weight by your activity level factor to determine the number of calories you should eat a day to maintain your current weight. (To lose a pound a week, you'll need to cut about 500 calories a day.)

_____ X _____ = _____
(A.L. factor)   (weight)   (calorie need)

For example: A 140-pound woman with a light activity level needs 1,960 calories a day to maintain her current weight.

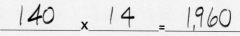

$$140 \times 14 = 1,960$$

If you're trying to lose weight, keep in mind that women shouldn't eat fewer than 1,200 calories a day, and men shouldn't eat fewer than 1,500 calories a day.

3 | determine how many carbs you need

The chart below assumes you need 50 percent of your calories from carbs. (Work with a registered dietitian to determine the best carb targets for you. According to the American Diabetes Association and the American Dietetic Association, carbohydrates can vary from 40 to 55 percent of total calories.)

Carb choices are foods that contain about 15 grams of carbs per serving. For example, 8 ounces of milk has 12 grams of carbs per serving and would count as one carb choice. You'll find the number of carbs listed on nutrition labels of your foods.

Calories	Grams of Carbs	# of Choices
1,200	150	10
1,500	185	13
1,800	220	15
2,000	250	17
2,200	275	19
2,400	300	20
2,800	350	23
3,000	375	25
3,200	400	27
3,400	425	28

4 | look at the fiber content of your food

If the food you plan to eat contains more than 5 grams of fiber, subtract the number of fiber grams from the total grams of carbs. For example, if a can of chili contains 24 grams of carbs and 9 grams of fiber per cup, count the serving as 15 grams of carbs, or one carb choice.

5 | spread your carb choices throughout your meals

If you want to eat five carb choices for breakfast, you could have 4 ounces of orange juice (one carb choice), two slices of whole wheat toast (two carb choices), ¾ cup of Cheerios with 8 ounces of milk (two carb choices), and a cup of black coffee (which has no carbs).

6 | check your blood sugar

Check your blood sugar before your meal and two hours after your meal and write down the results, along with what you ate. Making a record of what you eat and the way your blood sugar responds will help you make the best food decisions. Everyone's body will respond differently to the amount of carbs eaten, so it's essential that you find out how many carbs work for you throughout the day. Checking your blood sugar isn't necessarily something you have to do every day forever, but do it for several days to get a feel for how your body responds to your meals. Your target blood sugar levels should fall within these ranges:

Fasting or before your meals:
   90 to 130 milligrams per deciliter (mg/dl)
Two hours after the start of your meal:
   less than 180 mg/dl
At bedtime: 100 to 140 mg/dl

7 | make adjustments

If your blood sugar levels are too high two hours after a meal, try getting some exercise or adjusting your meal. Take a walk after eating to see if the levels go down, or trying taking out a carb choice. If that doesn't work, consult your health-care provider. Perhaps a medication adjustment will help.

8 | stay consistent

Eat your meals at around the same time every day. Skipping meals or varying the amount of carbs you eat at different meals from day to day will make it harder for you to control your blood sugar levels.

made with real fruit, and a handful of frozen mango chunks. Heat over medium heat until it forms a sweet glaze, and then drizzle over grilled salmon.

Throw thick slices of pineapple or peach on the grill. Brush them first with a little olive oil so they don't stick. Yum! Fruit has never tasted so good. You can even serve these for dessert.

Have a main dish salad once a week and give it the works. Put the same ol' vegetables in your salad every week and sooner or later you may be more inclined to toss it into the garbage disposal than savor every bite. Get out of the rut by trying new ingredients, such as spicy hearts of palm or artichoke hearts from a can, sweet and juicy raw jicama slices, steamed broccoflower heads (those chartreuse green cauliflowers you see at the store), nutty bean sprouts, steamed and marinated chayote squash (a Latin American squash with a citrus tang), or sautéed varieties of exotic mushrooms. Include a protein food such as beans or grilled chicken breast.

Try a new shape. Buy precut vegetables or cut them yourself into new shapes and you may find that you want to eat more of them. Carrot chips have a crunch that make you feel a little like you're eating potato chips. Cut zucchini or summer squash into long strips and grill. Imagine they're French fries!

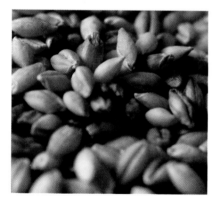

Use barley instead of white rice. For most people, barley raises blood sugar less than rice does (assuming you eat the amount of barley that you'd eat of rice), so consider it your new rice. (Test it and see for yourself!) Serve it with stir-fried vegetables, add it to soups and stews, toss it into your bean salad, or make it as a side dish. High in soluble fiber, it's a lot like oatmeal in the way it reduces cholesterol levels and the risk of heart disease.

Savor the sweetness of roasted veggies. Bring out the sweetness of vegetables such as eggplant, onions, peppers, zucchini, and summer squash by brushing them with olive oil, sprinkling with salt and pepper, and roasting in a 400°F oven until soft. On the grill, add firm vegetables such as eggplant, onions, and peppers right to the grill for 10 to 15 minutes. For softer or smaller vegetables like sliced zucchini, tomatoes, and carrots, use a metal grilling basket or grate and grill for 6 to 8 minutes.

Use veggies as fillers. Don't confine vegetables just to the side of your plate. Throw in a couple of handfuls of frozen peas and carrots to your rice or couscous during the last five minutes of cooking. Add chopped onions and spinach to meat loaf or hamburgers made with lean beef. Stir chopped peppers and mushrooms into canned or bottled spaghetti sauce. Add cooked collard greens, mushrooms, and onions to stuffing. Rub the fuzziness off of the stalks of okra, wash, slice, and add to soups, stews, and casseroles.

Give veggies more flavor by steaming them in chicken broth. Instead of adding water to your steamer or saucepan, add chicken or vegetable broth. You'll add flavor without fat to zucchini, cauliflower, carrots, sugar snap peas, and other veggies.

Save the water from steaming. After steaming your vegetables, pour the water into a covered jar and keep it in the fridge to use for broth the next time you make soup. The antioxidants from vegetables help stave off complications from diabetes, including problems with kidneys and eyes, and they may even help prevent the disease in the first place.

Think bean filling when you're itching for enchiladas. The next time you have Mexican night, skip the beef or chicken and fill your enchiladas and tacos with beans (not refried). For an easy meal of enchiladas, drain and rinse canned black beans and add them to a skillet with onions, mushrooms, and other vegetables. Add enchilada sauce and serve in whole-wheat tortillas with low-fat cheese.

Toss a five-minute bean salad. Choose three or four kinds of canned beans—such as garbanzo, black, kidney, navy, black-eyed, or waxed beans—and drain and rinse well to get rid of some of the salt. Then toss with chopped red onion, red pepper, and some vinaigrette-style salad dressing. Use about 1 tablespoon of dressing per ⅓ cup bean salad.

Replace white potatoes with sweet potatoes. Sweet potatoes raise blood sugar less than white potatoes do. If the sweet potato is large, cut in half and share one potato between two people. Be sure to eat the skin for its fiber.

Pair strawberries with wine or vinegar. A half cup of strawberries drizzled with balsamic vinegar or soaked in white wine makes for a sweet, indulgent-tasting dessert while satisfying about 75 percent of your daily vitamin C requirement. And like other berries, strawberries contain powerful antioxidants that help protect your body from the ravages of high blood sugar.

Have fruit for dessert. Fruit is, after all, nature's candy. So on those nights when you eat dessert (we suggest once or twice a week), try a roasted plum, a half cup of berries with yogurt on top, or a fruit crisp or crumble (go heavy on the fruit, oats, and cinnamon and very light on the sugar and butter).

"Bake" an apple in your microwave. Just core an apple, sprinkle the inside with cinnamon and a touch of sugar, and microwave for 3 minutes or until soft.

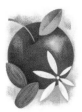

Berries contain powerful antioxidants that help protect your body from the ravages of high blood sugar.

diabetes-friendly snacks

"Don't eat between meals." If you've ever heard that advice, you might want to take it with a grain of salt. If you go more than four or five hours between meals, a mid-afternoon snack might be just what the doctor ordered to help you keep your blood sugar steady. Snacking is also important if you're taking medication that could cause a blood-sugar low between meals. Discuss with your doctor or a registered dietitian what snacking approach is right for you.

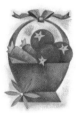

Nuts are packed with protein and "good" fat so they don't raise blood sugar nearly as much as crackers or pretzels.

Keep your snacks to 150 calories or less. The danger of snacks is that they can become more like extra meals if you go overboard. First, make sure you're truly hungry—and not just bored or stressed or craving chocolate—before reaching for a snack. Then limit yourself to 150 calories per snack. This will help keep your snacking "honest." After all, it's hard to find a candy bar with only 150 calories. And if you're hankering for a candy bar, but a healthier snack doesn't appeal, you're probably not truly hungry.

Beware of low-fat snacks. Studies show that people tend to eat about 28 percent more of a snack when it's low-fat because they think they're saving on calories. But low-fat snacks such as cookies only have about 11 percent fewer calories than their full-fat counterparts. Stick to the same amount you'd eat if you thought the snack was full-fat.

Plate your snacks. Eat straight out of the bag and you're guaranteed to eat more, whether it's chips, pretzels, or cookies. Instead, put a small portion on a plate, seal up the bag and put it away, then sit down and enjoy your snack.

Grab the whole bag. A single serving bag, that is. You're much more likely to stop after one serving if you don't have to measure it out yourself. If paying more for extra packaging that will eventually clog landfills bothers you, separate your snacks yourself into reusable single-serving containers when you get home from the grocery store so they're ready to grab when you're ready to eat them.

Pour a handful of nuts. Almonds, walnuts, pecans, peanuts, and cashews contain the healthy monounsaturated fats that lower cholesterol and reduce the risk of heart disease. And because they're packed with protein and "good" fat, they won't raise blood sugar as much as crackers or pretzels do. Because many nuts are high in calories (almonds are the lowest), stick to an ounce, or about the amount that will fit in the palm of your hand.

Have a few whole-grain crackers with peanut butter. You'll eat more protein and fewer carbs than if you have a bigger pile of crackers with no peanut butter, and your blood sugar won't rise as much.

whip it together! Cheesy Zucchini Bites

When you're hankering for a tasty, cheesy snack, pop these in the oven and enjoy a low-carb, healthy treat.

Cut a **zucchini** into ¾-inch slices and scoop out some of the inside flesh. Add ½ teaspoon crumbled **blue cheese**, top with a **tomato** slice, a sprinkle of **Parmesan cheese, basil,** and **pepper**. Bake at 400°F for 5 to 7 minutes, or until the cheese is melted. One zucchini bite has only 1 gram of carbohydrate, 19 calories, and 1 gram of fat.

Snack on raw veggies. Get in an extra serving of vegetables by nibbling on grape tomatoes, carrots, red and green peppers, cucumbers, broccoli crowns, and cauliflower. Eat them plain or dip them into nonfat yogurt, a light salad dressing, or hummus (stick with 1 to 2 tablespoons' worth).

Spread some black bean salsa over eggplant slices. The salsa has only about 15 grams of carbs, 80 calories, and 1 gram of fat.

Sip a small cup of vegetable soup. Cook non-starchy vegetables such as spinach, onion, celery, green beans, and squash in some vegetable or chicken stock. It's filling, full of veggies, and low in carbs.

Indulge in a few decadent bites. Have a snack of three dried apricots, a small piece of dark chocolate (about the size of a Hershey's miniature chocolate bar), and three walnuts or almonds, suggests Vicki Saunders, RD, who teaches nutrition education programs at St. Helena Hospital in Napa Valley, California. Savor every nibble!

Blend a fruit smoothie. Combine half of a chopped banana, ¾ cup non-fat plain yogurt, and a non-nutritive sweetener, and blend until smooth.

Freeze grapes and peeled bananas. Seal them in a sandwich bag and throw it into the freezer. Once frozen, they're a refreshing and healthy treat. You can eat 20 red seedless grapes and still consume only 100 calories.

Eat an apple—and the skin. An apple with the skin contains about 3 grams of fiber. The skin packs a double whammy, carrying healthy soluble fiber that helps to lower cholesterol and prevent heart disease and antioxidants that fight free radicals and lower the risk of diabetes complications.

Try low-fat string cheese. Each one contains only 80 calories. These are one of the few portable goodies rich in sugar-steadying protein.

Have your chocolate "bar" frozen. By that we mean enjoy a frozen fudge pop. They taste delightfully chocolatey but contain only about 80 calories.

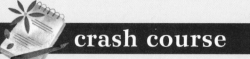

exercising with a kitchen chair

With only the help of a straight-backed kitchen chair, you can get a pretty good workout while you wait for the water to boil or the roast to come out of the oven. Do these moves every time you cook dinner and you'll be more limber, with a greater range of motion, and a bit stronger in no time flat. You may even feel calmer and more relaxed afterward—and be less likely to overeat at dinner!

1 | arm lift

Sit in the chair and extend your arms to either side at shoulder height, palms facing forward. Slowly, over the space of 5 seconds, **raise** your arms until your hands meet over your head. Hold this position for 5 seconds, and then spend 5 more seconds returning your arms to the original position. Repeat 5 more times.

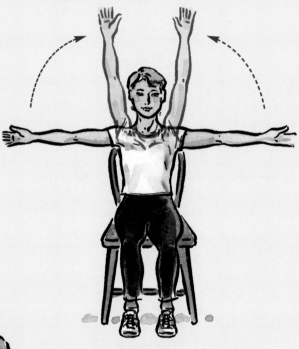

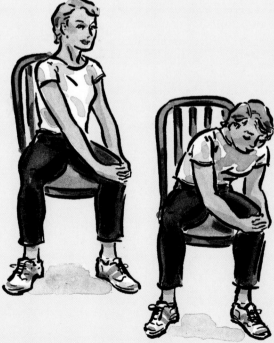

2 | back stretch

Sit in a chair, with your feet flat on the floor. Lace the fingers of your hands together and place them across the front of your right knee.

Lean as far toward your right knee as you can, breathing out as you do, and then **return** to an upright position. Spend 3 seconds leaning forward and 3 seconds returning. Repeat 4 times, then switch sides.

3 | leg lift

Sit with your feet flat on the floor. Slowly, over the space of 5 seconds, **lift** your right leg until it extends straight forward. Hold for 5 seconds, slowly **lower** it back down. Repeat 9 more times, then switch legs.

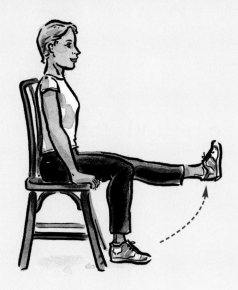

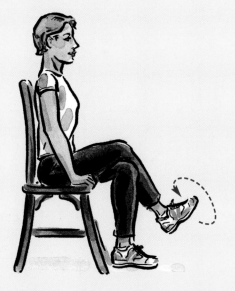

4 | foot circles

While sitting, **cross** your right leg over your left knee. Over a period of 4 seconds, **move** your right foot to the right and **draw** a large circle. Repeat 9 times, then switch feet.

5 | quarter squat

Stand behind the chair and place your hands on the top of the chair back. **Squat** slightly, lowering your hips about 4 inches, making sure your knees don't extend beyond your toes. Spend 2 seconds lowering yourself and 2 seconds standing erect again. Repeat 7 more times.

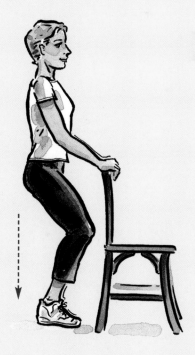

(continued on page 60)

6| knee lift

Turn sideways to the chair back and place your left hand on the chair back.

Keeping your back straight, slowly **raise** your right knee as high as it will go, then slowly **lower** it again. Still holding the chair back with your left hand, perform the exercise with your left leg. Do the exercise 5 times with each leg.

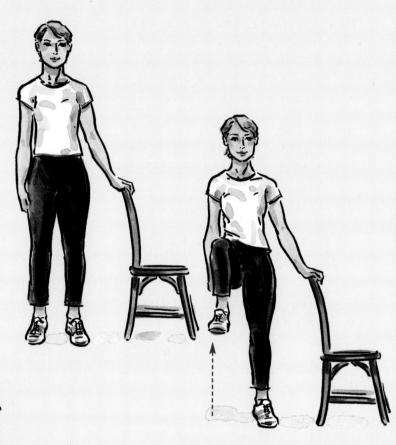

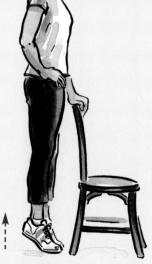

7| heel raise

Stand behind the chair with your feet 4 inches apart, your left hand on the chair back, and your right hand on your hip. **Raise** onto your toes over 2 seconds, and then **lower** back down over 2 seconds. Repeat 9 more times.

special mission: curb your carbs

Too many of the carbs we eat today are the kind that raise blood sugar too high too fast—muffins, cookies, white bread, and other baked goods made with white flour; easily digested starches such as potatoes; and refined grains such as white rice. Eating too many of these foods increases insulin resistance and makes it harder to control your blood sugar, so take aim.

Skip the dinner rolls. Bread isn't bad for you, especially if it's whole grain. But if you had a sandwich at lunch or toast with your eggs at breakfast, that's probably all the bread you need for the day.

Nix the tortilla for a lettuce leaf wrap. Wrap the lettuce around canned tuna or salmon, shredded carrots, diced celery, and pepper slices.

Hold your sandwich together with eggplant slices instead of bread. Broil the eggplant until brown, then add sliced mozzarella and tomato.

Mash cauliflower instead of potatoes. Add steamed cauliflower to your blender and puree with enough fat-free milk to make it velvety. Then drizzle with olive oil and season with salt and pepper.

Make cauliflower "rice." Using a food processor, shred cauliflower until its texture resembles rice, then lightly steam. Add this cauliflower "rice" to recipes that call for cooked rice.

Indulge in parsnip and carrot "fries." Cut down the length of parsnips and carrots to make long, thin strips of the vegetables. Place on a baking sheet, drizzle with olive oil, sprinkle with salt and pepper, and roast in a 400°F oven for about 40 minutes.

Replace potato salad with coleslaw. Coleslaw makes a great side dish—cabbage is low in calories and high in fiber. For the dressing, whisk together ⅔ cup fat-free sour cream, ⅔ cup plain nonfat yogurt, ¼ cup cider vinegar, 1 tablespoon of low-fat mayo, and 4 teaspoons sugar. Toss with 8 cups shredded red and green cabbage, 2 ounces blue cheese, 4 Granny Smith apples cut into wedges, and 2 slivered red bell peppers.

Cut your pasta in half. Serve yourself half of a cup of pasta instead of a whole cup and bulk it up with sautéed peppers, mushrooms, spinach, or other vegetables.

Feel a carb craving coming on? Drink a glass of water and wait 15 minutes. If you're still craving a particular food, put one serving on a plate and sit down at a table to eat it. When you're done, get out of the kitchen. It will keep you from overeating without feeling deprived.

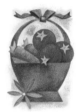

Cabbage is incredibly low in calories and high in fiber.

at the table

In general, people are on better eating behavior when they're in public or with a group of friends or business associates. For example, you're less likely to finish off your meal in record time. When you're at home, practice these tips at the table to help yourself slow down, eat more moderate portions, and even sneak in some extra vegetables.

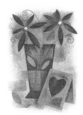

Dieters say that looking at themselves reminds them of their goals.

Get out Mom's china. Smaller plates mean you'll naturally eat smaller meals, and plates from the 1930s and 1940s were as small as five to six inches in diameter. A typical plate today? Ten to 12 inches. If you'd rather save the china for special occasions, use salad plates instead and save the dinner plates for company.

Banish the television from the kitchen and dining room. It's too easy to fall into mindless eating when you're in front of the TV. Another good reason not to watch: Studies show that the more time people spend in front of the television, the more likely they are to be obese.

Hang a mirror near where you dine. Watching yourself eat makes it much harder to gorge on food or eat too fast. Also, dieters say that looking themselves in the eye helps remind them of their goals.

Set a 30-minute timer before taking your first bite. Then don't take your last bite until it goes off. It takes about 20 minutes to feel full after eating, so taking it slowly will allow your brain to catch up to your stomach and turn off the urge to keep eating.

Skip "family style" meals. Setting out a heaping plate of spaghetti and meatballs will only tempt you to overindulge, so serve food on individual plates (with the possible exception of vegetables) and in moderate portions.

Encourage extra servings of vegetables by serving them in a big bowl or platter. No matter what vegetable you're serving for dinner, put out a lot and let people help themselves—and go back for seconds.

Put out a plate of raw veggies. If your family tends to mill around the table just before dinner is served—or if you yourself feel the need to nibble before the food hits the plates—have carrot sticks, cucumber slices, string beans, cherry tomatoes, or any other raw veggies out where everyone can easily reach them. Picking at them can substantially lower your consumption of the more calorie-dense main course.

Leave two bites on your plate. You can save more than 100 calories a day if you don't take those last two bites at lunch and dinner.

chapter three

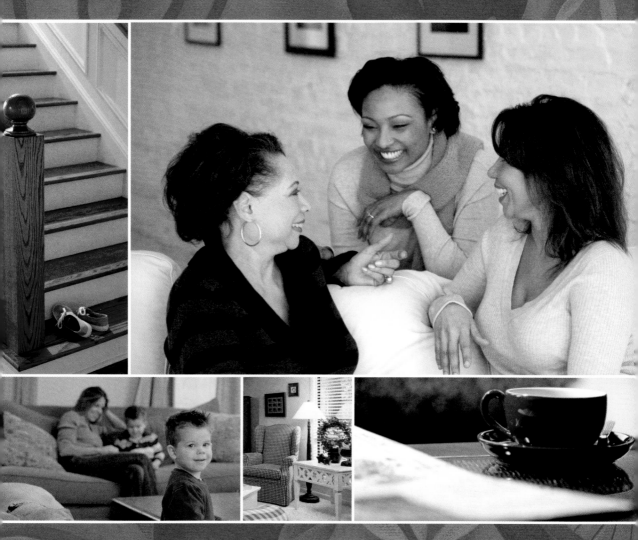

in your living room

Of all of the places we spend our time, this is where we do most of our living. Tweak a habit here and there and maximize your fun *and* your health.

better TV: "watching" your waistline

Few modern conveniences have done more to damage the health of humankind than the television. We barely move a muscle while we're glued to the screen, and images of fatty and sugary foods tempt us at every commercial break. The next time you hit the living room couch and press the remote control "on" button, keep these tips in mind.

Make a to-do list for commercial breaks. Ten minutes before the start of your favorite show, make a list of five two-minute projects that you can accomplish during the commercials. Your list may include things like dusting the living room blinds, sorting through the magazine rack, watering plants, and giving the cat her flea treatment. Gather all of the materials you need for these projects, and keep them at the ready. Accomplishing these little tasks will keep you moving around the house—and the distraction will keep you away from junk food in the kitchen.

Disable, then hide, your remote control. Take a trip down memory lane, back to a time when televisions didn't have remote controls. Changing the channel and adjusting the volume got you up and about, didn't it? Pulling the batteries out of your television's remote control and hiding it in a drawer on your entertainment center will get you off the couch and on your feet. And while you're up, you may remember to engage in another non-television distraction.

Pull the plug on "TV dinners." If you love hauling your dinner into the living room to dine in front of the television news or a game show, break the habit. Researchers have discovered that the more television people watch while eating, the less fruits and vegetables they consume. Scientists theorize that this is because television typically hypes diet-wrecking foods, which influences on-the-spot eating decisions on the part of the viewer.

Keep snack foods as far as possible from your couch. Storing chips, cookies, or other snacks in a cabinet near the television makes it way too

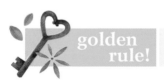

golden rule!   Use Exercise Toys While Watching TV

Use the time in front of the tube to get some exercise, even if it's mild exercise. Break out your elastic exercise bands (see page 214) to do some simple strength training, or jump on the stationary bike or treadmill while you enjoy your programs—even folding laundry is better for your body (and your household) than being a couch potato.

easy to eat junk food without even thinking. If you store them at the back of the pantry you'll at least have to get up to get them—and passing the fruit bowl on the counter will remind you that an apple would be a better snack.

Nibble on baked, not fried, chips. If you just can't make it through your late-night talk show without a handful of salty potato chips to snack on, switch to the baked variety. Whereas one serving of regular potato chips contains 150 calories and 10 grams of fat, the same serving of the baked variety contains 110 calories and 1.5 grams of fat. It's not just potato chips that are available baked—it's easy to find baked tortilla chips and other snacks, too. Just remember to eat no more than you would if the snacks were fried.

Brush your teeth after dinner. Many successful dieters confess that teeth-brushing is their secret weapon to weight loss. Once you've eaten your evening meal, get those pearly whites minty fresh. You'll be less likely to mindlessly dig into a gallon of ice cream or chew on pretzels while you're watching TV.

Keep your hands busy. Sometimes we end up smoking or nibbling on fattening snacks because we just want to keep our hands busy. Put those idle hands to work by doing needlework, stringing beads, cutting coupons, or knitting while you're on the couch. The more engrossed you become in your hobby, the less likely you are to reach for a snack—you don't want crumbs on your crafts!

Roll back your viewing hours. Scientists say that the more people watch TV, the more they eat. If you'd like to whittle a few chocolate chip cookies out of your diet, here's a simple way to do it: Study each night's schedule, identify one show you would have watched, and cross it off of your evening's agenda. Instead, walk down the street and throw pebbles into the creek, or call a friend you haven't heard from in months. Exercise and social connection will do your body and soul much more good than a television crime drama and the extra snacking that comes with it.

Have a joke for dessert. If you're going to watch television after dinner, punch up a comedy rather than a drama. Japanese scientists discovered an interesting thing about people with diabetes who laughed their way

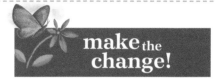

make the change!

The habit: Watching less television.

The result: Lower body weight.

The proof: Researchers from the United States Department of Agriculture surveyed more than 9,000 adults about their eating and television viewing habits. Adults who watched less than one hour of TV daily (only 15 percent of those surveyed!) consumed on average 1,896 calories per day, compared to 2,033 calories among those who watched more than two hours a day (nearly 60 percent of those surveyed!). What's more, the men in the second group were 22 percent more likely to be overweight or obese than those in the first; the women in the second group were 36 percent more likely to weigh too much. The researchers concluded that watching a lot of television or videos intrudes on time you might otherwise spend at physical activities. Also, people tend to consume more high-calorie snack foods while they're watching the tube.

whip it together! Crispy Cheese Chips

If you must have a snack in front of the tube, make it a healthy one! These treats pack a ton of crunch without the guilt that comes with chips and cookies.

Cut two 8-inch **whole-wheat tortillas** into 8 triangles. Coat a baking sheet with nonfat cooking spray. In a small bowl, combine 2 tablespoons **olive oil**, 1 finely minced **garlic** clove, and ½ teaspoon of dried **basil**. Brush this mixture over each of the wedges. Sprinkle ¼ cup grated **Parmesan cheese** over all wedges. Bake at 350°F for 8 to 9 minutes until toasted.

through a television comedy right after a meal: They had lower blood sugar than people who watched a humdrum lecture.

Juggle while watching the evening news. Stash three juggling balls or bags in a cabinet of your entertainment center. With your television tuned to the news, stand up, grab the juggling equipment, and practice your toss-and-catch through the broadcast. Not only will you impress friends at the next block party, but your goofing around will burn more than 270 calories per hour. You can buy juggling balls at toy stores, or use any balls that fit nicely into the hand and won't damage the floor or furniture when you drop them.

Hide resistance bands under the couch. These stretchy latex bands, sold in sporting goods stores and large department stores, can give just about any part of your body a great workout even while you're watching TV. Tie one end to the couch leg and the other end to your ankle, then try to straighten your leg for a good leg workout. Repeat 8 to 12 times, then switch legs. For more resistance band exercises, see page 214.

Watch a fitness show. If you're going to watch TV, why not get inspired by one of the "reality" shows in which people are charged with getting fit or losing weight? Better still, rent or buy an exercise video or DVD and pop it in. You can find all different types of exercise (aerobics, Pilates, yoga, tai chi, stretching, belly dancing, and more) for just about every fitness level—even seated workouts for seniors.

hit the "off" switch

Even better than being active while watching TV is pulling the plug alto-gether. Yes, there *are* other things you can do in your living room! Activities that allow you to interact with friends and family members—such as a live-ly game of cards—are easy ways to decompress while keeping your mind working. And if you just can't be compelled to get off the couch, why not at least invite your sweetheart to join you? If your intimacy leads you to the bedroom, all the better: Sex is a renowned stress reliever. One scientif-ic study demonstrated that when couples have sex, their blood pressure returns to normal more quickly the next time they encounter a stressful sit-uation—and the effect lasts for as much as a week.

Create a game cabinet. Appoint yourself your household's "game master" and stock a shelf or cabinet with board games and other amusements. Set a night every week on which you flick off the television, invite some friends over, and play dominoes, Monopoly, Scrabble, poker, Parcheesi, or some other mind-bender. You'll get a mental workout, engage in some friendly competition, and have some sugar-lowering laughs.

Put together an enormous jigsaw puzzle. There's something Zen-like in the quiet, contemplative process of slowly building a jigsaw puzzle. You turn your atten-tion for hours on the minute detail of a painting or photograph, and gradually the image materializes before your eyes. Buy the biggest jigsaw you can handle—some have thousands of pieces—and devote a card table or other surface to this low-tech, stress-relieving pursuit. You'll happily let the television stay dark for the evening (and, if the puzzle's big enough, many evenings to come). It's just as good a solitary activity as it is fun for the whole family.

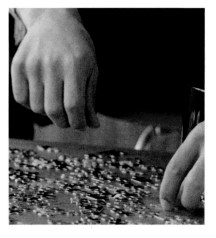

Organize your family photos. What household doesn't have a mountain of snapshots that need to be organized? Dispensing with this source of clutter will be stress relief in itself, but you also will get an emotional lift when you glimpse the photos again. If you don't already have a photo organization system, try this: Find a shoebox or another box that's the right width to accommodate snapshots. Use cardboard rectangles as dividers between categories of photos. (You can also buy photo boxes with these dividers.) Write a category label across the top of each divider ("Martha," "Christmas," "Family," and "Pets," for instance). As you go

(continued on page 70)

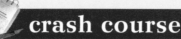
have a ball while exercising

They may look like giant toys, but stability balls, sold in most sporting goods stores, provide a fun way to exercise indoors. The inflatable balls are used primarily to strengthen back and abdominal muscles, though they can also improve balance and flexibility. They're lightweight enough to stow in a closet, but some people like the balls so much that they make them fixtures in the living room. Here are a few exercises to get you started.

1 | hip lift

Lie on your back on the floor, with your hands palms-down at your sides and your heels placed on the stability ball.

Tighten your abdominal and buttock muscles as you slowly **lift** your hips into the air until your body makes a straight line. Hold for 3 seconds and slowly **return** to the starting position. Repeat a total of 10 times.

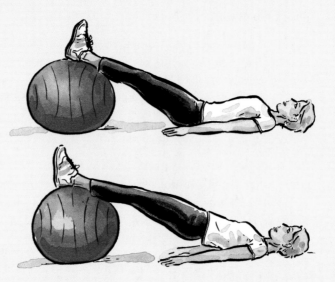

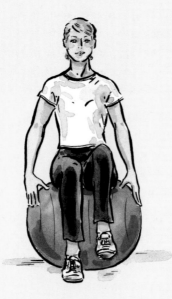

2 | balance challenge

Sit on top of the ball with your feet flat on the floor, hip-width apart. Place your hands on the ball at your sides. Hold your back straight and pull your abdominal muscles in. Now **lift** your left foot 6 inches off the ground, hold it there for 5 seconds, and **return** to the starting position. Repeat with the right foot. Do the exercise a total of 5 times with each foot. For more of a challenge, place your hands behind your head.

3 | back extension

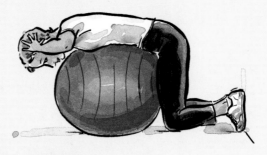

Start on your knees, with your feet against a wall and the ball on the floor against the front of your legs. Lean forward onto the ball, raising your knees 4 inches off the floor. Place your hands on either side of your head to the side of your head, fingertips near the temples and elbows straight out to the side.

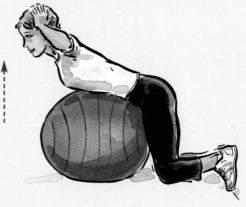

Raise your upper body until your back is straight, pause, then **lower** your body again until your chest rests against the ball. Repeat a total of 5 times.

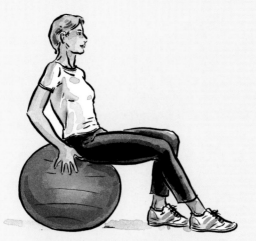

4 | forward walk

Sit on top of the ball with your feet flat on the floor. Place your hands on the ball for balance, or place one hand against a wall if you need the support.

Slowly **step forward**, letting the ball roll up your back until your shoulder blades are on top of the ball and your legs are bent at right angles. Slowly **step back** to the starting position. Repeat a total of 3 times.

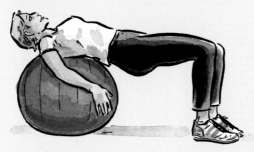

TRAINING TIP choose the right ball for your height

If you're 4 feet 11 inches to 5 feet 4 inches, you'll probably want a 55-centimeter ball. If you're 5 feet 5 inches to 5 feet 11 inches, go with 65 centimeters. Taller folks should look for a 75-centimeter ball. Your hips should be level with or just slightly higher than your knees when you sit on it.

through each envelope of photos, slide the very best into an album, file other photos you want to keep into the appropriate category in your shoebox, and throw out the rest.

Play a game of "musical massage" with your partner. Load your CD player (one that accepts multiple disks) with music that gets you "in the mood." You make half of the selections, and your partner makes half. Light a candle and turn out the lights. Turn on the music, and be sure to set the player on random mode, also known as "shuffle." The rules of the game are simple: As long as a song you selected is playing, you are giving the massage. As long as a song your partner selected is playing, your partner is giving the massage. "Play" continues until the two of you think of something else to do.

Go on a romantic "campout" tonight. For an adventurous approach to intimacy, "camp out" in the living room for the night. Move the coffee table and other obstructions out of the living room to create a wide open space. Bring into the room any large potted plants. Get two battery-powered camping lanterns (fuel-powered lanterns are a no-no inside) and zip two sleeping bags together. Put a nature sounds CD on the stereo. Have a bowl

whip it together! Sweet Balsamic Onion and White Bean Spread

You and your friends have planned an impromptu card game—you need a healthy snack to serve, and quick! This spread does the trick. Serve with whole-wheat crackers or crunchy veggies.

In a skillet, heat 1 teaspoon of **olive oil**. Add ½ cup chopped sweet **onion** and sauté for 5 minutes. Add in 2 teaspoons of **balsamic vinegar** and continue to cook for 2 to 3 minutes. Remove pan from heat and set aside. In a blender combine the following:

1 can (15 ounces) drained **navy beans** or **chickpeas**

2 minced **garlic** cloves

1 tablespoon finely minced **red onion**

1 teaspoon minced fresh **thyme**

1 teaspoon minced fresh **oregano**

2 tablespoons fresh **lemon juice**

2 tablespoons **olive oil**

Salt and **pepper** to taste

Add the onion mixture to blender and blend again until smooth.

of berries and a couple of steamy romance novels at the ready. Slide into the giant sleeping bag with your partner. Take turns feeding each other berries and reading passages from the novels to each other.

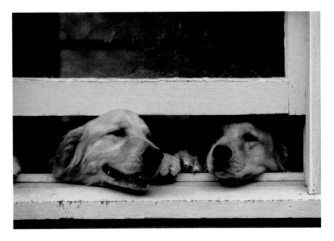

Challenge your dog to tug-of-war. If you have a large dog, you can get a pretty good workout this way. Teach Spot to tug on one end of a length of rope while you hold the other. Holding your elbow at your side, slowly raise your hand to your shoulder and lower it again (the bicep curl motion). When your bicep (the muscle on the front of your upper arm) tires, exercise the tricep (the muscle on the back): Starting with your arm straight down at your side, move your hand backward, pulling on the rope, and then return your hand to the starting position. When your arm tires, switch to your other arm and repeat both exercises.

Play hide-and-seek with Fido. Give your dog a command to stay in the kitchen, and then go hide elsewhere in the house—behind the couch, behind a door, or in a closet, for instance. Then call your dog. If he obeyed the "stay" command until you called and was able to find you, give him a treat. A few rounds of hide-and-seek will reinforce your pet's training and give you a bit of exercise to boot.

Offer 15 minutes of "fetch." Identify a stretch of the room that's at least 10 feet long, preferably 15 or 20 feet. Stand at one end of this "runway," and toss a toy or ball for your dog (or cat, if it's willing to play). Choose an item that won't harm the floor, walls, or furniture—preferably one that makes noise. Most pets will get the hang of this game quickly and return the ball to you again and again. Every time you receive the ball, do a knee-bend as you take it from the dog's mouth. Your dog may be doing more work, but the throwing, bending, and reaching is doing you some good as well.

Play "fish" with your kitty. Go to the pet store and buy a "cat-fishing" rig—a yard-long plastic rod with a string on one end that dangles a feathery toy. When you get home, stand in the living room holding the rod and letting the toy rest against the floor. Your cat will creep toward the toy. Test your own reflexes against your kitty's: Can you snatch the toy away just before she pounces? You can alternate between tapping the toy on the floor and dangling in the air to give Muffy her exercise.

burn calories at home

You *know* that exercise is a fundamental part of managing diabetes, but excuses to avoid huffing and puffing are more plentiful than daffodils in the spring: It's too rainy to go for a walk. It's too cold. The mall, with its sheltered walkways, is too filled with teenagers. With some basic at-home equipment, the living room can be your own private gymnasium. (Or put the equipment in the family room or basement.) You can also get exercise without equipment just by keeping up the house.

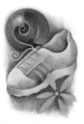

Scientists say upbeat music makes exercisers work harder.

Vow to keep clothes and junk from cluttering the treadmill. A treadmill is exercise equipment, but if you treat it like a clothes rack or an extra shelf, you're hardly likely to walk on it—so don't clutter it up in the first place! When your exercise equipment is at the ready for a workout, you have one less excuse standing between you and your health goals.

Jump on your bike or treadmill before 10 a.m. Researchers say that people who get their workouts done early are more likely to stick to their exercise plans because the task is completed before other obligations distract you. There's an added health bonus, too: Exercise produces feel-good brain chemicals called endorphins, which will give you a lift that will last the better part of the day.

Move your feet to a high-energy beat. Before you jump on your treadmill or stationary bike, turn on some high-energy music. Scientists say exercisers work 5 to 15 percent harder when they're listening to upbeat tunes.

Give yourself a "thrill" while working out. Web sites for large book retailers, such as Amazon.com, sell audio CDs of contemporary thrill novels (some libraries have them, too). Pop your purchase into your disc player, raise your right hand, and take this oath: "No matter how engaging I find this story to be, I will only listen to this recorded book while I am walking on the treadmill in the family room." You'll find yourself actually looking forward to your workout—it's the only way to find out what happens in the next chapter!

Make a weekly date with your vacuum cleaner. Not only will this help ensure that your feet are protected from debris, but vacuuming also burns nearly 240 calories an hour. And your flooring—whether it's carpeting, wood, tile, or vinyl—will last longer and look nicer when it's free of abrasive, ground-in dirt.

make your living room an oasis

Stress and high blood sugar go hand in hand. Instead of seeking food or mindless television as solace for your tension and anxiety, try one of these soothing approaches. Making even one small change in your daily routine can add up to a calmer outlook and feeling more in control of your life.

Compose a heartfelt letter on pretty stationery. In an era of cell phones, e-mail, and instant messaging, penning a letter and hand-addressing the envelope is a gratifying return to simpler ways, not to mention a wonderful way to keep in touch with those you love. And what a treat it will be when the return letters start outnumbering the junk mail and bills in your mailbox. Get started by keeping these items in the drawer of your coffee table or end table: a comfortable pen that you love to write with, stationery that's appropriate for all occasions, your address book, and stamps.

Make afternoon tea a daily ritual. Teatime is relaxing, and anything that keeps stress hormones from raising your blood sugar is a blessing. But did you know that both the black and green varieties of tea help protect your vascular system? In one study, people who were heavy tea drinkers were 44 percent less likely to die after they had a heart attack than people who did not consume tea. And tea consumption appears to help prevent health problems in the first place—including heart attacks and diabetes. Scientists believe that tea keeps your blood vessels supple, helps to prevent artery blockage, and discourages blood clots. If you sweeten your tea, try a sugar alternative such as a non-nutritive sweetener or stevia to reduce the carb content.

Get a chair that rocks. Buy a rocking chair for your living room and sit in it, saving the recliner for a guest. Screen one of your favorite classic movies, and keep the rocking chair going for the duration. It may not seem like

(continued on page 76)

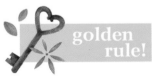

golden rule! Keep Your Shoes On

Your living room may have wall-to-wall carpet, but that doesn't mean you should stroll around barefoot and fancy free. Protecting your feet is too important for people with diabetes, particularly if the condition has left you with reduced feeling in your feet, which makes it more diffi-cult for you to tell if your feet are injured. Even on that plush carpet, it's still possible to step on sharp objects or stub a toe. If you have hard flooring in your living areas, wear shoes or slippers that provide cushioning under your feet and support around the ankles.

meditation

When you hear the word "meditation," a slight frown probably crosses your face. Isn't meditation a "fringe" activity for hippie-types who like to burn incense? In short, no. It's simply a way to distract your mind for a few minutes from your churning thoughts and your daily worries—no incense or "lotus" positions required. And you can do it from your easy chair.

For a person who has diabetes, there are very real physical benefits to meditating. Especially if you're feeling stressed, anxious, or out-of-control, it can help you calm your mind and body, reducing your levels of stress hormones. This in turn can lower your blood pressure and boost your immune-system activity (helpful because in people with diabetes, wounds often take longer to heal). Daily meditation can even reduce the risk of heart attack and stroke.

Meditation isn't a way to escape your life; it's a way to let yourself feel more comfortable with it—and who doesn't want that? Follow these tips to get started.

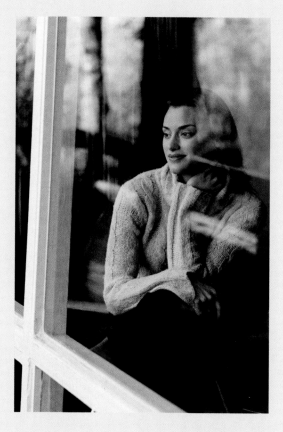

1 | easy steps to get ready

Wear comfortable clothes. Put on loose clothing that does not pull, squeeze, or bind you. Make sure that your belt and shoes are not too tight or causing you discomfort.

Pick just the right spot. Comfort is key. So is serenity—be sure to choose a quiet spot where you'll be free from noise and other external distractions. The easy chair in your living room is a fine candidate if you're not too slumped in it—a straighter posture may promote mental alertness and lessen your chances of falling asleep. It also allows for freer, easier breathing. Some people prefer sitting on the floor, perhaps near an open window.

Have a clear view of the clock. You will want to know when your meditation time is over, so position a clock within sight of your meditating spot. Your watch won't do because you don't want to have to lift your arm and focus on the small numbers to read the time.

Choose a word. Call it a mantra if you wish, but really it's just one calming word (preferably just one or two syllables) that you can focus on while you meditate. Words like "peace" and "joy" are good candidates. Another school of thought is to pick a sound like "ohm" so that you're focusing on your breathing rather than the meaning of the word.

2 | focus on two simple things

Once you're ready, distract your mind for 10 to 15 minutes. You may close your eyes or leave them open—it's up to you. If you prefer your eyes closed, you will need to open them occasionally so you will know when your 15 minutes have passed. Focus on just two things:

Your breathing. Breathe deeply and pay attention to the air as it enters and leaves your lungs. It doesn't matter whether you breathe through your mouth or your nose.

Your word or sound. Repeat it to yourself in your head each time you exhale. If any other thought starts creeping into your head, consciously direct your mind back to your word or sound and to your breathing. Keep everything else outside the bubble of peace that you're in. When your breathing becomes completely relaxed, you won't even hear yourself inhale or exhale. Your goal is to be awake and alert, but not at all tense.

3 | time's up. now what?

That felt good, didn't it? Well, meditation feels better and better over time. Try doing it every day. And don't give up: It could easily take eight weeks for you to get totally comfortable with meditation. Eventually, you'll learn to stop "talking to yourself" in your head, which can be difficult. And you'll slip into a state of alert relaxation faster and faster. Once you have the hang of it and meditation feels natural, do it three times per week, 15 minutes per session.

Besides helping you manage your diabetes, meditating regularly can make you a calmer, more efficient person, and it should improve your interactions with others.

4 | guided imagery: another way to relax

Think of guided imagery as a wonderful vacation without the hassle of security checks and baggage claim. Led by a voice on an audiotape or CD, you relax while the person leads you through a series of comfortable mental experiences involving all of the senses, beautiful vistas, and welcoming people. Your body responds as if what you're imagining is real. Tapes are designed for specific purposes, such as reducing stress, managing pain, losing weight, and easing insomnia. Look for them wherever you buy music or books on tape.

A related practice, called visualization, requires no tapes, just your imagination. Here you picture a relaxing scene using all your senses. For instance, imagine yourself on a sunny beach. See the seagulls diving for fish, feel the wind on your face and the sand beneath your feet, smell the ocean air, listen to the crash of the waves, even taste the salty water in your mouth when you dive under.

much effort, but over the course of a nostalgic evening, that's more foot and calf stretching than you realize!

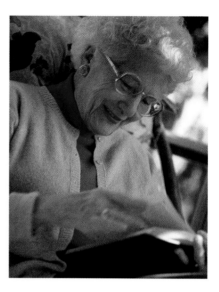

Turn some pages and climb Mount Everest. Reading is relaxing—and it can also be motivating. How many of those books by your easy chair have some element of health, sports, or physical activity? If your answer is "none," visit the library and ask for recommendations that will put you in an active, healthy mindset. Try Babe Ruth's biography, or *Into Thin Air*, written by a climber who survived a disaster on Mount Everest. Or check out a travel guide and plot out an active vacation. Also look for inspiring tales of people who have overcome major obstacles; they will make yours seem infinitely small and highly manageable.

Keep your curtains open while it's light outside. Natural light boosts your levels of the feel-good brain chemical serotonin. Not much sun outside your window? You can also buy bulbs that simulate natural sunshine; their blue wavelength, which is missing in conventional light bulbs, makes all the difference.

Put noises on "mute." Blaring, jarring noises make your living space more stressful. Outfit your television, computer, and audio systems with headphones so that their users won't fill the house with unwanted sound. Carpet your living room if possible, and favor upholstered furniture. If you and your partner use noisy appliances frequently, strike an agreement with him or her to establish some quiet hours each evening. If noise from the outside is a real problem, consider installing noise-reducing windows.

Warm up your living space with autumnal colors. Decorating your home in warm yellow, gold, orange, and red tones will warm up your mood, too. Rehabilitation facilities use this golden color scheme to keep patients upbeat and happy—and it's no surprise that it works, because it mimics the effect of sunlight.

chapter four

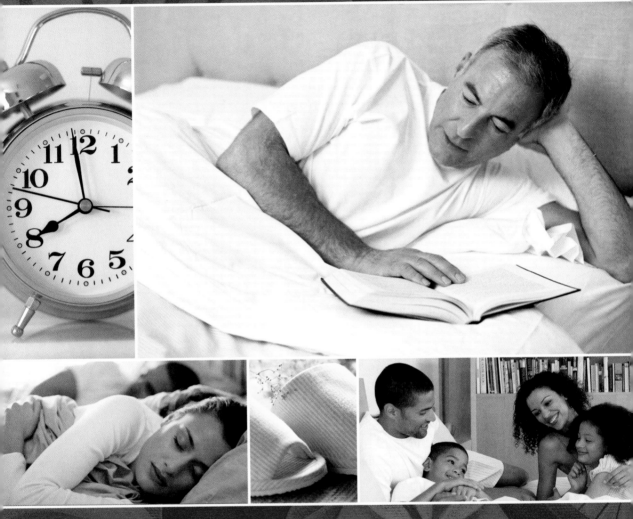

in your bedroom

The bedroom brings it own set of pleasures, from luxurious sleep—critical to good blood sugar control—to stress-relieving, calorie-burning private time with your partner. Here, discover how to make your room a haven for body and soul.

getting quality sleep

Long-term lack of sleep can make blood sugar harder to manage by reducing your body's sensitivity to insulin, the hormone that moves glucose out of the bloodstream and into your cells. It can also boost the risk of a long list of medical problems that people with diabetes are already prone to, including obesity, high blood pressure, heart attacks, and strokes. If you don't feel well rested when you wake in the morning, rally yourself to action. The payoff of deep, luxurious slumber is well worth the effort.

Go to bed and wake up at the same times every day. Your body likes predictable cycles, so give it the gift of a sleep schedule that it can count on. This means going to bed at the same time every night and waking at the same time every morning, even on weekends. You'll fall asleep faster, and you'll be more likely to get the right amount of sleep each night.

If you do want to sleep in, do a quick test. Controlling your blood glucose and sleeping late on your day off can seem downright incompatible for people who are on insulin. But with a little effort, you can do both (remember, sleep late on weekends only if you don't suffer from insomnia). The night before your "sleep late" day, set the alarm for a relatively early time—say, 6 a.m. When it goes off, check your blood glucose. If it's high, talk to your doctor about taking two units of fast-acting insulin. If it's normal, take a unit or two of regular insulin. If it's low, drink a glass of juice or milk. Then jump back into bed and close your eyes for a few more hours, secure in the knowledge that your blood sugar is under control.

Aim to get at least 30 minutes of exercise a day, five times per week. Physical activity is a boon to so many body functions, and sleep is one of them. That gentle fatigue you get from exercise will set your body up for a

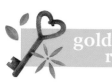

golden rule!

Get at Least Eight Hours of Sleep Every Night

Can poor sleep lead to poor blood sugar control? Experts think so. Researchers at the University of Chicago studied 161 people who have type 2 diabetes. Only 6 percent of the patients were getting at least eight hours of sleep a night, and 70 percent of them reported routinely getting poor-quality sleep. Lack of sleep or poor quality of sleep was closely associated with higher A1C scores, a measure of blood sugar levels over the long term.

"We've known for some time that skimping on sleep can impair glucose tolerance for healthy people," said researcher Kristen Knutson. "Now we have evidence connecting chronic partial sleep deprivation and reduced blood-sugar control in patients with diabetes."

good night's rest. So for the sake of shut-eye—on top of all of the other health benefits—stick to your exercise regimen. Just be sure to stop exercising several hours before bedtime.

Wind down three hours before bedtime. As you wind down in the evening, reduce your activity level the closer you get to bedtime. Three hours before lights-out, cease vigorous physical activity. One hour before bed, engage in a quiet activity that relaxes you—that might be taking a bath, stretching gently, meditating, praying, reading, or listening to pleasant music. Twenty minutes before bedtime, dim the lights. By the time you pull your covers to your chin, your eyelids will be drooping.

Check your blood sugar regularly. Many people with diabetes have their blood sugar checked when they visit the doctor two or three times a year, but they don't do their own checking in the interim—a bad idea. Either high or low blood sugar levels can affect your sleep. If you're not feeling fully rested in the morning, commit to regular self-checking so you can take steps to stabilize your blood sugar between doctor visits.

Either high or low blood sugar levels can affect your sleep.

In the middle of every night this week, check your blood sugar. For one week, set your alarm for 3 a.m. and check your blood sugar each time. If you find consistently normal readings, that should set your mind at ease. If you find that your blood sugar is below 75 mg/dl when you check it at 3 a.m., eat a snack. Keep graham crackers in the drawer of your nightstand for this, and have a bottle of water handy to wash them down. If you find an ongoing pattern of low blood sugar in the middle of the night, talk to your doctor about the possibility of adjusting your nighttime insulin dose or the snack you eat (if any) before bed.

Nod off in total darkness. Close your window coverings so that they block out as much light as possible. Even better, purchase shades or drapes that are specially designed to block out sunlight. In addition, make sure that there are no glowing electronic devices in your bedroom, like televisions, alarm clocks, or nightlights that might distract you from sleep.

Keep a flashlight on your nightstand. When you wake during the night needing a trip to the bathroom, you don't want to wake your partner by turning on the light. But stumbling around in the dark just invites a stubbed toe. A flashlight directed at the floor just in front of you will escort you safely to the bathroom and back.

Let nighttime noises fall on deaf ears. Trying to sleep in a noisy atmosphere is tough, and it may even raise your blood pressure. So it's worth investing a little time and money to make your bedroom as quiet as possible. If your partner watches the evening news in bed while you're trying to nod off, buy him a set of cordless headphones. If his snoring keeps you awake, invest in some earplugs. To block out street noise, you could pop in a compact disc that plays nature sounds or buy a "white noise" machine, which generates a dull yet calming sound that covers other noises. Or simply turn on a fan and be lulled to sleep by its low whirring sound.

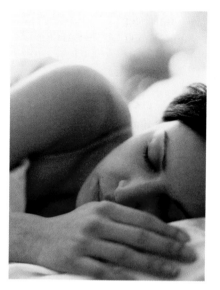

Turn down the thermostat before you climb under the covers. Researchers at the University of South Australia have found that insomniacs have a higher core body temperature than those who don't have trouble sleeping. The university's Centre for Sleep Research experts say that the body starts to lose heat between 60 and 90 minutes before you fall asleep. If you're not sleeping well, you can help your body wind down by keeping your bedroom moderately cool—say, between 68°F and 72°F, or cooler if you prefer. (Ask your spouse to consider wearing warmer clothes to bed if he or she finds your ideal temperature too brisk.)

If you've had a beer, have a healthy snack, too. If you've enjoyed so much as a glass of wine or beer in the hours leading up to your bedtime, do a quick check of your glucose levels. If your blood sugar is low, have a small snack if you need one before crawling under the covers. Alcohol makes it difficult for your body to recover from low blood sugar; having a bite to eat will moderate its effects.

Stop drinking two hours before bedtime. To reduce your nighttime urination, and therefore interrupted sleep, don't drink liquids of any kind in the two hours before you go to bed. When you put less fluid in the "pipeline" before you hit the sack, there will be less fluid building up in your bladder during the night.

If you have chronic pain, invest in a high-quality mattress. A mattress that conforms to your body may give you the extra help you need to sleep through the night. Prepare to pay a lot more for these mattresses. If cost is an issue, look for a conventional mattress that's supportive and firm.

Sleep on a thin pillow if you're a back sleeper. If you like to sleep on your back, you should sleep on a thin pillow. Pillows that are too thick will compromise your body alignment and cause pain in your neck. If you prefer to sleep on your side, a thick pillow will provide better neck support and therefore better sleep.

Test yourself for sleep apnea. Does your partner say you snore loudly or seem to be holding your breath while you sleep? You might have sleep apnea, a malady that interrupts the rhythmic breathing that other sleepers enjoy. Sleep apnea can aggravate diabetes-related conditions like high blood pressure, obesity, and impotence. It also raises the risk of heart disease. If you sleep alone and always wake up exhausted, set up a noise-activated recorder before you go to bed to help you rule out sleep apnea. If you suspect you have it, talk to your doctor. A continuous positive airway pressure (CPAP) machine, connected to the sleeper by a mask and hose, is often the answer.

Let yourself see the sunshine. According to the National Sleep Foundation, sunlight (or other bright light source) is the "most powerful regulator of our biological clock." Seeing sunlight helps to regulate the body's wake-sleep cycle. When it's exposed to sunlight, your body knows to inhibit production of the sleep-inducing hormone melatonin, and when night falls, melatonin goes into high production. If you're homebound and not sleeping well, lack of sun exposure could be the reason.

Make your evening cup of joe a decaf—or a cup of herbal tea. Reducing or eliminating your caffeine intake will go a long way in helping you get better sleep. Check the labels on your herbal tea and soft drinks (including colas, root beers, orange sodas, Mountain Dew, and other sodas), and avoid anything with caffeine in the six hours before you retire for the evening.

Limit naps to 30 minutes or less. If you're napping during the day and not sleeping well at night, you just might be napping too much. The American Academy of Sleep Medicine recommends that you keep daytime naps to less than an hour; 20 to 30 minutes is ideal. Finish your nap by 3 p.m.

Screen Your Feet for Nerve Damage

The Lower Extremity Amputation Prevention (LEAP) program will send you a free kit for assessing loss of feeling due to nerve damage in your feet. It includes a tool that's designed to apply precisely 10 grams of pressure against the foot. If the screening reveals loss of feeling at any of the spots indicated in the instructions, alert your doctor. You can find information on the LEAP program on the Internet at www.hrsa.gov/leap, or by writing to LEAP, Health Resources & Services Administration, 5600 Fishers Lane, Rockville, MD 20857.

Talk to your doctor if you're feeling blue. The American Diabetes Association reports that people with diabetes are at a greater risk for depression than people who do not have diabetes; the reasons for this are unknown. Depression can interfere with sleep. If you find yourself lying awake early in the morning and feeling hopeless or "down," talk about it with your doctor. It's possible that treatment for depression, which may include medication, psychotherapy, or both, will put you on the path to better sleep.

Write down your to-do list before you hit the sack. How many times do we lie down and drift off only to bolt awake because we forgot to pay a bill or make an appointment? Keep a notebook at your bedside table so that you can write down things that you have to do the next day, or any other worries that have been nagging you throughout the day, to free your mind for sleep.

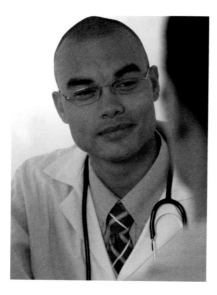

Tell your doctor if you have stinging pain in your legs. If a painful sensation that feels like bees attacking your feet is keeping you awake at night, ask your doctor if you have neuropathy (nerve damage) in your legs. Treatments for another condition, restless leg syndrome, are frequently advertised on television, but don't assume that's the problem—neuropathy is different. Prescription drugs including certain antidepressants and anticonvulsants can provide relief for this sleep-robbing malady, or your doctor may recommend over-the-counter painkillers such as aspirin, acetaminophen, or ibuprofen. Some people find that walking regularly or wearing elastic stockings helps, too.

Rub on pepper cream to relieve foot pain. Creams that contain capsaicin, the "hot" ingredient in hot peppers, may provide relief for people who have foot pain caused by nerve damage. Rub some onto your feet three or four times a day. Initially, the cream will provide a warm sensation. Over several weeks, the nerve pain will subside. Be sure to wash your hands immediately after applying the cream, or use protective gloves to apply it, and make sure it doesn't come in contact with your face. If you really want to turn up the heat, ask your doctor about a prescription-strength capsaicin cream.

creating a stress-free oasis

You spend about a third of your life in the bedroom, so why not make it a comfortable, soothing refuge? Remember, reducing stress helps reduce high blood sugar, since stress blocks the release of insulin. Here are a few tips to help you transform your bedroom's atmosphere.

Clear your room of clutter. Smooth, clean surfaces act as balm to your brain, so clean off the dresser surface, put away all the clothes strewn on your bedroom chair, and buy a bookshelf for that stack of books collecting dust.

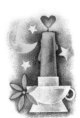

Color thera-pists say blue hues have calming and relaxing effects.

Once a week, put fresh flowers on your dresser or nightstand. A study at Kansas State University found that female office employees felt more relaxed when they were working near a vase of flowers. Just imagine how nice it would feel to *sleep* near one.

Scent your room with essential oils. In aromatherapy, a number of scents are recognized as particularly useful for reducing stress. There are several easy ways to introduce these scents into your bedroom. One is to buy a light bulb ring (a device that you set onto a cold light bulb), add a couple of drops of essential oil, and turn on the lamp to let the oil warm and scent the air. Another is to buy or make potpourri, a collection of dried herbs treated with essential oils. Or mix in a spray bottle 2 ounces of water, plus a drop or two of your favorite oils, and use the scent as an air freshener. Relaxing scents include bergamot, chamomile, lavender, lemon, marjoram, neroli, opopanax, orange, sandalwood, valerian, and ylang ylang.

When choosing bedroom hues, go with blue. Scientists say that the color blue affects the autonomic nervous system—the part that operates without your conscious control—to lower heart rate and blood pressure and slow breathing. Proponents of color therapy say that blue has a calming, relax-ing effect and helps lull you to sleep. If the room is due for a fresh coat of paint, go azure. If not, sprucing the room up with sky-colored blankets, pil-lows, and rugs will also do the trick.

Try a few feng shui tips. Feng shui aims to achieve harmony between your spiritual self and your physical environment. In this ancient discipline, proper positioning of elements of a room creates the desired energy flow and balance of forces. Practitioners recommend that you position your bed on the opposite side of the room from the bedroom door—not directly in front of the door, but diagonally across the room from it; position the bed so that when you lie in it, a window is to your right (to feed you positive energy when you wake up); and keep desks and computers, along with their work-related energy, out of the bedroom.

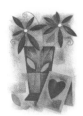

Sex can act like insulin, lowering your blood sugar.

diabetes and your sex life

Making love with your partner is a wonderful activity for your relationship and for your health. And people who have diabetes can enjoy fully satisfying sex lives, if they understand a few things about how diabetes affects the body. A frank talk with your doctor or your partner might be all that you need to do to make your romantic encounters more successful and enjoyable.

Use exercise to increase your libido. Here's further motivation to get your recommended daily dose of movement: Both men and women with diminished sex drive will benefit from routine exercise, experts say. Exercise improves your blood flow, which will improve the function and sensitivity of your sex organs. Stronger muscles, better aerobic capacity, and an improved self-image also will enhance your experience in the bedroom.

Check your blood sugar before making love. If your blood sugar tends to drop during physical activity or at nighttime, having sex in the evening can present a challenge. Before things get too heated up, check your blood sugar so that you're sure of your status. If your blood sugar is at the normal level or is already on the low side, you may need to adjust your insulin or eat something before or after sex—a robust session could make you hypoglycemic. If you have an insulin pump, consider unhooking it during sex.

Be careful if you're making love after you drink. Alcohol and vigorous sex both lower blood sugar, and combining the two could cause a dangerous low. Be sure to monitor your blood glucose if you're having "a glass of wine and thou."

Seek a "bonus round" of sex. If your doctor says your body can handle the physical activity, ask your spouse for one extra session of sex per week or per month, depending on how active you already are. On average, people burn 250 calories per hour during lovemaking. This aerobic "workout" will do your cardiovascular system a lot of good, and it's one less bad TV show the two of you will be watching.

If your libido is flagging, ask yourself two questions. First: Does your reduced sexual desire apply to all situations at all times? If so, review with your doctor the possible medical sources of your diminished sex drive. Medications you're taking or hormone problems could be the culprit. If the answer to the first question is "no," ask yourself: Does the strength of your sex drive depend on the situation? Perhaps you have little desire for sex with your partner, but you find other people attractive and get satisfaction from masturbation. If so, marital or psychological counseling could help.

Massage your partner tonight, and get a massage tomorrow night. The added relaxation may help to reduce your levels of stress hormones, which can drive up your blood sugar. And who know where a massage might lead? Even if it leads nowhere, this kind of touch is a nice way to connect with your spouse and show you care. A bonus for the massage giver: Because massaging someone takes force (more than you may realize), your hands and arms get some exercise.

Be especially touchy if you or your partner has nerve damage. It's rare, but in some cases nerve damage reduces sensitivity in the genitals in people who have diabetes. Often you can compensate for this with additional gentle touching in the right places. A vibrator might help as well.

Report pain during sex or cloudy urine to your doctor. High blood sugar compromises the body's ability to fend off bacterial invasion. If you feel pain during sex (especially for women) or have urine that's clouded or bloody, a burning sensation when you urinate, or constantly feel the need to urinate, talk to your doctor. You may have a urinary tract infection. Refrain from sex until the problem is resolved.

Don't be afraid to use lubricants. Vaginal dryness is common among women who have diabetes, and this is a simple problem to fix. Keep water-based lubricants in the drawer of your nightstand, each of them a different color, scent, or flavor. Some also warm when they make contact with skin. The variety will add a degree of sensuous play to your love life, which can be a bonus if you or your partner has a flagging sex drive. Stick to water-based lubricants. Oil-based lubricants (such as petroleum jelly) can damage condoms and lead to bacterial infection.

Prevent surprise pregnancies. These aren't a good idea for women who have diabetes. If you're pregnant and your blood sugar isn't under control, you run a high risk of birth defects or miscarriage. Your birth control options are the same as for people who do not have diabetes. However, if

golden rule!   ### Discuss Sexual Problems with Your Doctor

Set bashfulness aside, and tell your doctor if your sex drive is significantly lower than it used to be. Hiding the problem can weigh on your mind, leading to self-blame and despair, making your sexual performance even worse. For a person with diabetes, a number of factors could be responsible for reduced sex drive. Your doctor will know how to identify potential causes and get you the appropriate care.

you use birth control pills, monitor your blood sugar closely, and ask your doctor whether you need to adjust your insulin or other medications. Birth control pills work by giving you hormones, and some hormones can raise your blood sugar levels. And remember, women who have entered peri-menopause and are having irregular periods can still get pregnant.

Ask your doctor or gynecologist about the best birth-control pill for you. Some types, namely monophasic contraceptives, which contain fixed amounts of estrogen and progestin, appear to keep blood sugar more stable than triphasic pills or progesterone-only pills.

Guard against yeast infections. Women who have diabetes are more susceptible to vaginal infections and should take special care to avoid them. Higher glucose levels in the vaginal lining, combined with moisture and warmth, encourages the growth of bacteria and yeast. The problem is particularly bad for older women because levels of protective estrogen drop around menopause. Bathe regularly and keep fecal matter away from the vagina. Keep the vaginal area dry, and avoid clothing that will hold moisture against you. Avoid harsh feminine products that invite infection, including douches, feminine sprays, and strong soaps. Regardless of gender, get your blood sugar under control and talk to your doctor about medicated ointments and creams that will clear up the problem.

To prevent bladder infection, urinate before and after sex. If you're a woman with damage to the nerves controlling your bladder (neurogenic

Is Your Menstrual Cycle Affecting Your Blood Sugar?

Your menstrual cycle might be complicating your efforts to manage your diabetes. Women build up high levels of estrogen and progesterone about a week before menstruation. Some scientists believe that these hormones interfere with insulin sensitivity in many women, most often making blood sugar run high, but sometimes causing it to drop. So take out your record of blood glucose readings for the last three months and mark the dates when your last three periods began. Were your blood sugar levels *high* a week before each period? If so, experiment with some countermeasures. Exercise more around this time and cut back on carbs, for instance. If you use insulin, ask your doctor if it's okay to slowly increase your dose a touch and back off again when your period starts. If your blood sugar tends to *drop* a week before your period, do the reverse: Temporarily exercise less, consume more carbs, and lower your insulin dose slightly if your doctor says it's okay.

bladder), urinate just before sex and within 30 minutes after having sex. This will reduce your chances of developing a bladder infection.

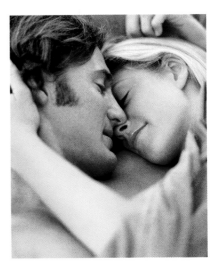

Don't be embarrassed to mention erection problems to your doctor. Impotence is sometimes an issue for men with diabetes. A wide range of factors—for instance, the nerve damage and blood flow problems that are common in people with diabetes—can contribute to erection problems, as can some blood pressure medications, taken by many diabetes patients. In fact, some 50 to 60 percent of all men who have diabetes and are over age 50 have erection problems. Your doctor won't be surprised to hear about your condition.

Identify the cause of your impotence before resorting to prescription medication. Some doctors are quick to write a prescription without taking a medical history and looking for underlying medical problems. Don't settle for a libido-enhancing pill as your first and only solution. By identifying the cause, you can find the best fix for you.

Take ginkgo biloba to give your blood flow a boost. This herbal supplement improves blood flow. Since an erection is basically a matter of hydraulics—blood flowing to the penis—taking gingko regularly could lead to better erections. Check with your doctor first, however, because this supplement can interact with other medications.

Test yourself for nighttime erections. Erectile dysfunction problems can be either physical or emotional. Here's an easy way to tell the difference. Before bedtime, wrap a small strip of paper around your penis and tape the ends together to form a band (don't put tape all the way around the penis). If the paper is broken in the morning, you probably had an erection. If a man is having erection problems during sex because of emotional issues, he will probably still have erections while he sleeps. The more scientific way to detect nocturnal erections is to have yourself monitored during sleep, either in a sleep lab or with a monitor you use in your own bed. If you are not having erections during sleep, your problems are likely physical.

Get a prostate checkup. If your sleep is frequently interrupted by trips to the bathroom, ask your doctor whether your prostate could be causing the problem. If your prostate is enlarged, it could be squeezing the urethra, the tube that urine passes through on its way out of the body. The result of that squeezing is that you feel as if you need to urinate more often.

treat your feet to TLC

Everyone gets a blister or callus now and then, but these little bothers are much more serious for people with diabetes, whose feet are particularly vulnerable to infection. Poor blood circulation (common with the disease) makes healing more difficult. And because of nerve damage, you might not feel sores, blisters, or cuts. Foot problems left untreated could even lead to amputation. So check your feet every night this week before you pull the covers back; the ritual will become second nature in no time.

Get your spouse to play "footsie" with you. There are many reasons that a person who has diabetes might have a hard time checking his or her feet thoroughly: Back problems, obesity, and arthritis may reduce the flexibility you need to inspect your feet closely. Diminished eyesight makes the task more difficult, too. In any case, enlist your spouse's help. The slight inconvenience that it might be to ask for someone's help is a lot better than finding out about foot injuries too late.

Keep a small mirror under your bed. It's pretty easy to see the tops and sides of your feet, but many people aren't agile enough to get a good look at the bottoms. If you have this quandary, buy a mirror that's about the size of a sheet of notebook paper and place it mirror-side up under your bed. At bedtime, use your toes to slide the mirror out from under the bed. Examine your feet in the mirror, and then slide the mirror back into its hiding place.

Keep your eyes open for irritations large and small. When you conduct your foot check, you obviously need to keep an eye out for open sores and cuts. Signs of infection in a sore include swelling, redness, drainage, oozing, or warmth. Call your doctor immediately if you see any of these symptoms around a sore, at the site of a splinter or cut, or around your toenails. Smaller signs of irritation need quick attention, too, including

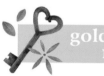

golden rule! ## Make Your Nightly Foot Check Automatic

When you slide into the car seat, you buckle your seatbelt without thinking. Make your foot check just that automatic. Every night when you pull off your shoes and socks, add one more little step to the undressing process: a thorough examination of your feet. Start with your toes, then do the bottoms, sides, tops, and ankles. Regularity is the key. You never know when a foot problem might surface, and catching it early will help you prevent serious complications. Amputation is not a negligible concern; people who have diabetes are 10 times more likely to require amputation than people who don't have diabetes.

redness, corns, or calluses. Pay particular attention to the toes and the ball of your foot when you inspect—that's where most foot ulcers develop.

Clean and treat minor scrapes and cuts right away. Wash your hands with soap and water. Then wash the wound with soap and water, rinse with more water, and pat it dry with a clean towel or paper towel. Dab some antibiotic ointment onto a cotton swab and smear a thin layer of the ointment onto the wound. (Don't apply the ointment with your finger.) Cover the wound with an adhesive bandage. If the wound does not look better within a day, or if you see signs of infection, such as swelling, redness, warmth, or oozing, call your doctor or a foot care specialist immediately.

Moisturize your tootsies. When you peel your socks off for the evening, check to see if tiny white flakes are falling to the floor. Those flakes are dry skin cells—if you see them, your skin is too dry, and you'll need to moisturize with a thick cream or lotion. If you don't moisturize, your skin could begin to crack, which will leave you vulnerable to infection. Pay particular attention to your heels and the balls of your feet, where dryness is most likely. Then tuck your feet into clean cotton socks, which not only keep your sheets from being streaked with lotion, they also seal the moisture into your skin. Applying moisturizer once or twice a day should be enough to keep skin from cracking.

Ask your podiatrist to trim your toenails at your next visit. Health-care experts are reluctant to have diabetes patients care for their own toenails because sharp clippers that are mishandled can cause injuries. Be honest with yourself: Can you reach your toes easily? Do you have a good set of toenail clippers? Will you take the time to do a careful and meticulous job of trimming? If not, ask your partner to do the task for you, or better yet, have your podiatrist do it.

If you do trim your own nails, use clippers designed for toenails. Toenail clippers are larger and have more leverage than fingernail clippers, so they can snip through thicker toenails without your applying excess pressure, which could lead to injury. Also, their blades are less rounded, making them more suitable for big ol' toes. You can purchase lever-style toenail clippers (which look like oversized fingernail clippers) or scissor-style clippers

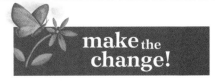

make the change!

The habit: Working with your health-care team to establish a foot care program.

The result: Reducing your risk of amputation by half.

The proof: Several large medical centers have established comprehensive foot care programs for people who have diabetes. These programs include treatment for foot problems, preventive therapy, patient education, referral to specialists, and referral to shoe fitters. With such programs, the centers found that they can reduce the numbers of amputations they perform by 45 to 85 percent. Ask your primary care doctor or podiatrist if there's a program at a hospital near you.

(continued on page 92)

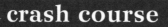
exercise in bed!

It's no fun getting out of bed only to be greeted by a chorus of complaining joints. Here's a set of gentle stretches and muscle-toning exercises you can do while you're still lying in bed. They should help reduce your stiffness and put you in the mood for the kind of physically active day that will help you control your diabetes. Start with just a few repetitions of each exercise and build up to the recommended number.

1| knee pull

Lie on your back. **Raise** your left knee and wrap both hands around the front of it. Gently **pull** your knee toward your chest and then **return** to the starting position. Repeat 2 to 4 more times. Then switch sides. This will stretch your lower back and the backs of your legs.

2| front stretch

Lie face down with your palms on the bed near your shoulders. Keeping your hips against the bed, **push** down to raise your head and chest. **Exhale** as you push, and stop when your elbows form a right angle. Hold for 5 to 10 seconds. Exhale as you **lower** yourself to the starting position. Repeat 3 to 5 more times. This will stretch the muscles in your abdomen, chest, and lower back.

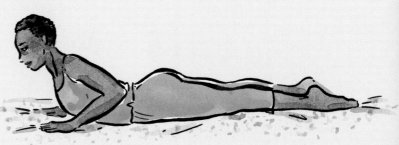

3 | thigh and groin stretch

Lie on your left side. **Move** your right leg behind you and **reach** back with your right hand to grasp the top of your right foot or ankle just behind the toes. **Arch** your back slightly and hold for 5 to 10 seconds. Repeat 2 to 4 more times. Switch to lying on your right side and repeat. This will stretch the tops of your thighs and the groin.

4 | tummy tightener

Lie on your back with your knees bent and your feet flat on the bed. **Lean** your head forward slightly and **reach** until your fingers touch your knees. Hold for 5 seconds, and **return** to the starting position. Repeat 9 more times. This exercise strengthens your stomach muscles.

5 | foot push

Lie on your back in bed with your feet flat against the footboard (or turn around and place your feet against the headboard). **Press** against the board with your toes, hold for 5 seconds, and **release**. Repeat 9 more times. This exercise strengthens your calf muscles and ankles.

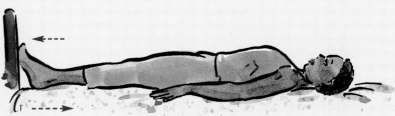

If you have reduced feeling in your feet, you might not notice a problem until it's too late.

(which look like mini-wire cutters). Nail files and emery boards are acceptable alternatives. Don't use conventional scissors or a knife, and don't tear, pull, or bite at your toenails.

Soften sharp toenail edges. When you trim your toenails, cut them so that they're flush with the tip of the toe, in a slightly curved shape that follows the shape of the toe. You often will see advice saying to cut toenails straight across, but this can leave sharp points on the sides of your nails that can cut into your skin or become ingrown. Use a file or emery board to smooth any rough or sharp spots.

Toss out your electric blanket. Don't bed down with any devices that will create extreme temperatures, such as electric blankets, heating pads, hot water bottles, and ice packs. With reduced feeling in your feet, you might not be able to tell when such items are overheating or over-chilling your feet or other body parts.

Slip into your slippers. If you have changed into your pajamas for the night but you're not quite ready to slip under the bedcovers, pull on a sturdy pair of nonskid slippers to protect your feet. Walking around barefoot is never a good idea for people with diabetes. Even if you are meticulous about housekeeping and won't risk stepping on something sharp, there are still plenty of ways in which you can stub your toe.

In the morning, check your shoes for lumps and debris. You know how cowboys camping in the desert shake out their boots in the morning in case a scorpion has crawled inside? You should do the same thing, even if you spent the night in the comfort of your bedroom. Before you pull on a pair of shoes in the morning, shake them out and run your hand inside to detect pebbles, other objects, lumps, or rough linings that could rub or injure your feet. Otherwise, if you have reduced feeling in your feet, you might not notice such a problem until it's done serious damage. Inspect the soles for any tacks you might have picked up, and make sure the soles are in good repair so your feet are getting proper support.

in the master bathroom

Yes, you can practice better diabetes management even in the bathroom! Decisions as seemingly minor as what kind of soap to use or how hot to run your bathwater really are important. Whether you're showering or treating your feet, follow these tips. Above all, vow to never, ever do "bathroom surgery" on your feet. Treating corns, calluses, and ingrown toenails is best left to the professionals. You could easily do more harm than good.

Use moisturizing bar soap. Wash your feet daily in water that's warm but not hot. Avoid liquid soaps; they are more likely to leave your skin dry, which can lead to cracking and therefore can leave you susceptible to infection. Also avoid exfoliating soaps, which can be too rough on your skin, and perfumed soaps, which cause skin reactions in some people.

Disconnect your insulin pump before showering. Even though pumps are water resistant, they shouldn't be put directly in the water. Use the disconnect port meant for swimming, bathing, and showering. Read the manufacturer's instructions or ask your doctor where to put the pump while you shower. For some pumps you can buy cases you can hang from a shower curtain hook.

Limit your soak in a hot bath to 20 minutes. If you're going to have a relaxing spell in a hot tub, a hot bath, a sauna, or a Jacuzzi, stay no more than 20 minutes, make sure the temperature is no higher than 105°F. (Be sure to clear this indulgence with your doctor in advance.) Excessively warm temperatures can aggravate cardiovascular problems, which are common among people with diabetes. If you're using insulin, a hot soak can increase the rate at which the body absorbs it, throwing off the timing of your blood sugar control. When you enter hot water, don't use your foot to test the temperature—if you have nerve damage, you might not realize your skin is scalding. Instead, dip a hand or elbow into the water, or use a bath thermometer.

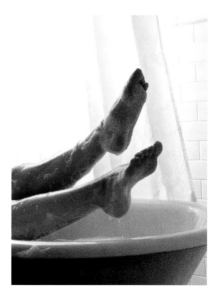

Pass on callus treatments. If you have diabetes, resist the temptation to use over-the-counter drugstore treatments on the calluses and corns on your feet. When you have reduced feeling in your feet, it's easy for such treatments to damage your skin without you knowing it. The active ingredient in both the liquids you dab on and the pads you apply is an acid that can eat away not only your dead skin, but your healthy skin, too. The resulting wound from the acid could take a long time to heal. Don't use pumice or a file on your calluses and corns, either; the risk of injury is too great, and such instruments aren't sterile. Ask your doctor or podiatrist to treat your calluses and corns so they don't have an opportunity to develop into sores.

Forget ingrown toenail treatments, too. Use of drugstore treatments for ingrown toenails also is not recommended. As with callus and corn removers, these products work by eating away the skin with acid, which puts you at risk for infection. Go to your podiatrist to have the ingrown toenail treated.

Treat athlete's foot with medicated cream. Athlete's foot is a fungal infection that people with diabetes can safely treat with drugstore products. Athlete's foot appears as red, itching, or cracking skin between the toes and on the bottoms of your feet. Treat this immediately, since the cracked skin can get infected. Apply athlete's foot cream twice a day. First wash your feet with soap and water. Dry them thoroughly, then rub the cream onto the affected skin. Call your foot care specialist if the athlete's foot hasn't cleared up within five days.

chapter five

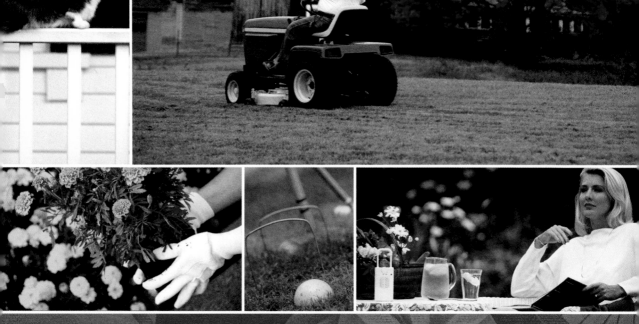

in your yard

Your yard is a veritable playground—a place to be active
and indulge in fun and games, to relax, to reinforce social
connections, and even to cook and enjoy healthy meals.
So step outside and let the outdoor living begin!

good times, good friends, and the great outdoors

When we speak of a home's "living" space, we talk about the square feet to be found inside. But oh, how much of the real living goes on in the yard! The next time friends and family come for a visit, invite everyone outside for some fun in the open air. Kick back and run around like a kid again—no "indoor voices" required.

Invite your neighbors to a croquet party. Besides being a great theme for a fun party, croquet offers health benefits: You'll get a little strength training by swinging your mallet, and ambling to and fro around your property will burn a few calories. Best of all, you'll have a few laughs and learn the latest gossip—and you won't have to dig into coffee cake to get it.

Hold an apple hunt. Before you have guests over for a backyard barbecue, buy two dozen apples of different varieties. Take a stroll around your property and find ingenious spots to hide the fruit. When guests arrive, give everyone shopping bags, and send them on an apple search. Have them bring their treasures to a picnic table, where you are prepared with a bowl of water for rinsing apples, plus a knife and cutting board.

Keep a badminton set handy and have it ready when family visits. For casual play, badminton requires little expertise, and it will keep everyone physically active and working as a team—and shift the emphasis of the visit away from food. Other easy games to keep in the garage include horseshoes, hula hoop, Frisbee, and ball-toss sets that use Velcro mitts.

Outfit your patio for outdoor eating. You'll need weatherproof furniture, an umbrella, and a grill. These basics will encourage you to spend time outdoors and dish up healthy "al fresco" meals like garden salads and grilled fish, chicken, and lean meats.

golden rule! Vow to Spend 20 Minutes a Day Outdoors

Spending time outdoors is good for you in so many ways. Getting outside for even a few minutes a day can reduce depression. It can also help you lose weight: Light activity outside (like gardening or washing the car) burns about six times the number of calories as watching TV. And unless you live in a very northern climate, a few minutes of sunshine during months when the sun is high in the sky helps the body make vitamin D. Deficiency in this vitamin predisposes people to obesity and increased insulin resistance.

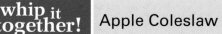

whip it together! | Apple Coleslaw

Why drown healthy, low-cal cabbage in fatty mayonnaise? Dressing your slaw up with apples, poppy seeds, and low-fat condiments yields heaps of flavor with fewer calories and less fat.

In a salad bowl, combine:

6 cups shredded **green** or **red cabbage** (or a combination of both)

2 diced, unpeeled **red** or **green apples**

2 peeled and shredded **carrots**

3 tablespoons **raisins**

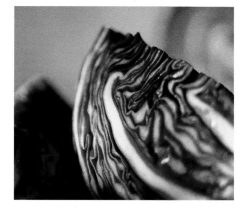

In a separate bowl, combine:

½ cup nonfat **mayonnaise**

¼ cup plain nonfat **yogurt**

2 tablespoons low-fat **sour cream**

1 tablespoon **poppy seeds**

2 teaspoons **apple cider vinegar**

1 teaspoon **honey** or **sugar substitute**

Salt and **pepper** to taste

Add the dressing to the vegetable mixture and toss well. Cover and refrigerate for ½ hour before serving.

Play hoops and sticks with the little ones. If you're old enough, you may remember the old hoop and stick game, and the fun you had chasing that rolling circle, tapping it now and then with your wooden wand. But to today's kids, the game's a jaw-dropping curiosity. Pick one up at a toy shop that specializes in nostalgic amusements, or search for one on the Internet. Hang it in your shed and whip it out the moment the grandkids start reaching for their headphones and electronic games.

Install a bird feeder. Watching birds is incredibly relaxing, and a feeder is what you need to attract them to your yard. Check a field guide to find out what kinds of birds you are likely to attract, and then buy a feeder and seed that suits their preferences.

Add a birdbath. Birds also need drinking and bathing water. Add four or five copper pennies to the water to block the formation of algae so you have to change the water less frequently.

ready, set, grill

Sure, firing up the barbecue or gas grill provides you with a sociable, relaxing time in the backyard, which is an instant stress buster. But it's particularly beneficial for people with diabetes because grilling happens to be a healthy cooking technique. Grilled foods typically don't require high-fat sauces or accompaniments. And much of the fat drips away and never makes it to your plate. Here are a few ways to make your outdoor cooking even *more* healthful.

Bypass burgers and fill the grill with seafood and lean cuts of meat. You don't have to gorge on fatty burgers and bratwursts just because you're cooking outside. Healthier choices include skinless chicken breasts, beef tenderloin or sirloin, and fish.

Disrobe your chicken. Or you can leave the skin on while it's cooking to seal in moisture, and pull it off afterward. It will save you a load of saturated fat—which hampers insulin sensitivity and increases the risk of heart disease—and calories.

Bathe meats in a vinegar-based marinade. A study conducted at Arizona State University found that eating 4 tablespoons of cider vinegar before eating a high glycemic-index meal (one that includes foods that tend to raise blood sugar quickly) lowered the effect of the meal on participants' blood sugar by about 55 percent. Low-fat Italian vinaigrette salad dressing with extra vinegar added will even do the trick. You also can experiment with your own marinades using vinegar, olive oil, wine, lemon juice, lime juice, garlic, and herbs.

Splurge on grilling lessons. Grilling may seem simple, and it is—if you know how to do it properly. You'd be surprised at how valuable even a few simple grilling secrets can be. Do you know how often to flip a piece of meat and when to do it? How to tell when the food is done without cutting into it? The more you know, the more fun you'll have. For a special event such as a milestone birthday or anniversary, consider hiring a chef to come to your backyard. He can whip up a meal for your party and work in a lesson. Ask him to focus on healthy foods that you don't know how to grill—say, salmon fillets, scallops, or pork loin. The more healthy dishes you're excited to cook at home, the fewer calories (and dollars) you'll waste at restaurants.

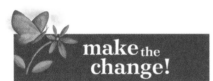

make the change!

The habit: Grilling fish instead of breading and deep-frying it.

The result: Less saturated fat and fewer calories consumed.

The proof: A 3.5-ounce serving of whitefish fried in batter contains 231 calories and 12 grams of fat, 3 of them saturated. But when you grill it naked, the same serving of fish contains only 112 calories and only 1 gram of fat (and no saturated fat). Making this easy switch cuts your calorie intake by more than half and cuts out the saturated fat, which hampers insulin sensitivity and increases the risk for heart disease.

whip it together! Balsamic Mustard Grilled Shrimp Kebabs

You can't go wrong with kebabs, which deliver maximum healthy flavor with minimum effort. Vary this recipe by substituting scallops, cubed chicken, or lean pork for the shrimp.

⅓ cup **balsamic vinegar**

2 tablespoons **Dijon mustard**

1 tablespoon **olive oil**

2 tablespoons **honey**

2 minced **garlic** cloves

2 minced **scallions**

1 pound peeled and deveined large **shrimp**

8 **cherry tomatoes**

8 **scallions**, white parts only, cut into 1-inch pieces

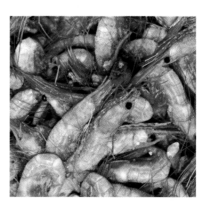

Combine the first 7 ingredients in a medium bowl. Cover and marinate for 1 hour. Drain the shrimp from the marinade. On a skewer, alternate shrimp, cherry tomatoes, and scallion pieces. Use 3 shrimp, 2 tomatoes, and 2 pieces of scallion for each kebab. Grill over high heat for 2 to 3 minutes per side or until shrimp are cooked through.

Skewer some squash, portabello mushrooms, eggplant, and zucchini. Many of your favorite fruits and vegetables will pick up an alluring new taste when grilled. Sliced squash, eggplant, bell pepper, portabello mushrooms, onions, tomatoes, pineapple, peaches, and apricots all fare well on a grill. Coat veggies with a little olive oil before adding to the grill. For small or thin slices that might fall through the bars of your grill grate, use skewers or special grilling baskets, which you can buy in home improvement and cooking stores.

Grill delicate foods in packets. Making dinner on the grill doesn't automatically mean charbroiled meat and corn on the cob. Packet cooking lets you cook all sorts of foods on the grill. Just center the ingredients on a large sheet of aluminum foil, add a little olive oil or broth, then fold up the sides, leaving some room for steam to circulate inside. Set the packets on the grill. This strategy works particularly well for delicate or quick-cooking foods, such as fish and boneless chicken breast. Even lean meats stay tender. Put out a variety of vegetables (bell peppers, onion, snap peas, corn, etc.) and seasonings and let each member of the family design his or her own packet.

put yourself to work

If you're going to exert yourself, you might as well get some fresh air and a beautiful yard in the process! Many people find yard work satisfying because you—and your neighbors—can immediately see the results. Set aside some of your "convenience" equipment in favor of some old-fashioned muscle power, and you'll burn even more calories while you work.

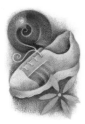

Washing your car burns 200 to 300 calories per hour.

Make appointments with yourself to spruce up the yard. Make a list of every yard and outdoor chore that needs to be done around your house. Break them down into 30-minute jobs. ("Mow front yard" and "Mow back-yard," for instance.) Some of these jobs will be seasonal, and others will be monthly or weekly. Store this file where you will be able to refer to it regularly and add to it as you think of more jobs. On the family calendar, schedule 12 to 15 jobs that are appropriate for the next month. You're more likely to keep appointments with yourself if you write them down.

Wash your car every week in good weather. As kids, there was no better household chore to tackle in the dead of summer than washing the family car: You got a chance to cool off with spray from the hose (and admit it, you horsed around with your siblings, too). Washing your own car today can be almost as fun, and with the prices of professional washes as they are, it's a real money saver, too. Hauling buckets of water, dragging the hose around your vehicle, and scrubbing and buffing your car's finish will burn between 200 and 300 calories per hour.

Shovel snow by hand. If you live in a snow-prone region and have a drive-way that's 50 yards long, okay, you need a snow blower. But many of us who have conventional driveways or a few square feet of asphalt to clear around a car that's parked on the street will get through the winter just fine with an old-fashioned, broad-bladed snow shovel. Even light show shovel-ing can burn more than 545 calories per hour, and your shoulder and arm muscles will get quite a workout. If that's too much of a challenge, use the

golden rule!   Bend with Your Knees

Gardening and other yard work can be awfully tough on your back. When you need to lift something, stand close to it and bend at the knees to pick it up. That way, your legs are getting a good workout, and you won't strain your back. Another way to protect your back is to carry a small stool with you to sit or lean on while weeding. You might also consider plant-ing a raised gardening bed.

snow blower on the driveway, but switch to a shovel for the sidewalk and front steps. Shoveling can be strenuous, even for very fit people, so check with your doctor before digging yourself out.

Skip the string trimmer. Unless you have a yard that rivals the grounds of Buckingham Palace, a power-driven string trimmer is probably more than you really need. Instead, tame the unruly grass blades that border your flower bed with a spring-loaded hand trimmer. Just be sure to keep the blades sharp, the mechanism lubricated, and wear work gloves to prevent blisters.

Rake your own leaves. Sure, leaf blowers might just be one of the best inventions out there, but they're so loud that some communities have banned their use. Do your ears and your neighbors a favor and cut back on your leaf blower use. If you have so many leaves that you can't handle them with a rake alone, walk the perimeter of your yard with the leaf blower and corral them toward the center of the lawn. Then complete the job with your rake. You'll still work up a sweat and burn nearly 300 calories per hour.

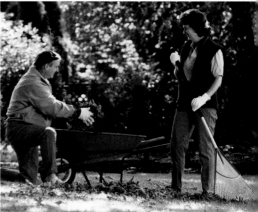

Trade in your riding lawn mower. You don't have to push very hard to guide a self-propelled non-riding mower, but the walking will provide a nice aerobic workout.

Swing an ax, and heat your home this winter. Don't let the firewood folks deliver a cord of pre-chopped logs to your backyard. That's robbing you of great arm, shoulder, and back exercise. Starting in mid-summer, chop your own wood for half an hour every weekend. By the time snow falls, your upper body will be toned, and you'll have the fuel to keep your home toasty.

Install your mailbox on the very edge of your property. Take down that mailbox that's right outside your front door—that's not getting you any exercise. Install your mailbox either at the very end of your driveway (or even farther out, if your property is expansive) and walk out for your mail each day. Once you're off your driveway, you may be inspired to take a turn around the block.

cultivate a gardening habit

Your yard does double duty as a gym and a relaxation spa when it contains a garden. In fact, studies find that gardening is one of the best activities around when it comes to preventing or improving chronic health conditions. Shoot for a minimum of 30 minutes of gardening (or other yard work) three to five days a week. You'll be controlling your diabetes and raising your property value at the same time.

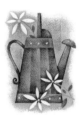

By hoeing, digging, and lugging the watering can, you'll be getting an excellent workout in the garden.

Pencil in autumn bulb-planting on your calendar. Take the family calendar, flip to one of the autumn months, and write "bulbs" on three back-to-back weekends. Plan for each bulb-planting session to last an hour. All of that digging will give you a week's worth of strength training for your arms and shoulders, and your flowerbeds will be the envy of the neighborhood when spring rolls around.

Be a hands-on sodbuster. When you start up a new garden, or you're preparing an old one for new planting, break the soil up yourself with a shovel. If you're particularly ambitious and your garden is too big to till in one session, break up the job into smaller sessions or go ahead and rent a tiller, which will still exercise your arms. In either case, wear gloves to prevent blisters.

Forgo poison and pull weeds by hand. Give the soil in your yard a break from weed-killing chemicals. Instead, pull the interloping plants out of the dirt by hand. All you need are gloves, a small weed-digging tool, a bucket or bag in which to discard the weeds, and perhaps kneepads. With your right hand, jab the weed-digging tool into the earth at the plant's base to loosen the roots, and then pull it out with your left. Every 10 minutes, switch hands. The activity not only beautifies your yard, it'll burn 306 calories per hour for a 150-pound person.

Plant a front yard flower showcase. Pick a flower bed in your front yard that's prominent on your property and visible from the street—this is where you will devote 75 percent of your flower-planting efforts. Now give that bed the full treatment: well-fertilized soil; a newly installed, handsome border; carefully scheduled watering; and flowers selected for color, height, and season-long blooming. By hoeing, digging, and lugging the watering can, you'll be getting an excellent workout in the garden, and you won't even notice. To top that, the neighbors strolling by will ooh and aah, and you may even strike up friendships that you wouldn't have otherwise.

Bring a radio outside and change up your tasks every four songs. Varying your activities will help you avoid putting too much stress on one set of muscles. For instance, you might start by pushing heavy wheelbarrow loads of mulch from your driveway to the backyard, then switch to watering flower beds.

Grow a healthier garden by keeping a compost pile. Compost piles are good for the environment because they return biological materials such as grass trimmings and banana peels to the soil. But that's not all—cultivating them can give you a physical workout, too. A compost pile needs to be turned periodically to keep the rotting process humming along, which requires a little hoeing, raking, shoveling, or pitch-forking. You can burn off 250 to 300 calories in just 30 minutes of pile-turning.

Turn off the sprinkler. The easiest way to water your garden is to set up a sprinkler, but that doesn't do your body any good. The next time you need to give your plants a lift, take a turn around the yard and aim the hose at each plant individually—not only will you be able to monitor each plant's progress more closely, but tugging and carrying the hose will do your muscles good. When this becomes easy for you, haul out the water can instead of the hose. You'll know that your strength has improved when you're able to fill the can all the way and carry it with ease.

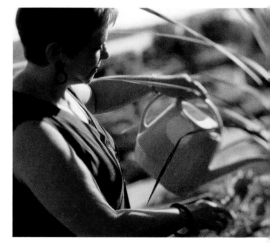

Plant your own "locally grown" vegetables. Veggies you grow yourself are as local, and as healthy, as you can get: You know that they're fresh as can be, and you know exactly whether pesticides or other treatments have been used on them. Successfully harvesting your own tomatoes, beans, lettuce, squash, and other vegetables is also a point of pride. You'll be so pleased with yourself for having cultivated them that you're more likely to cook them frequently and experiment with new recipes, and you'll make sure that they'll never go to waste.

Plant an herb garden. There's no better way to add big flavor to your meals than with fresh herbs, but they're awfully expensive at the grocery store. The solution? Grow your own. Culinary herbs tend to thrive in hot, dry conditions where nothing else seems to flourish. Try sage, oregano, thyme, rosemary, tarragon, and basil. For the most flavorful herbs, feed plants only with compost, and water them as little as possible. This encourages compact growth and intensifies the oils that give the herbs their fragrance and flavor. To dry the herbs, cut sprigs early in the morning, when the fragrances are strongest. Place them in a large paper bag (one for each type of herb), then put the bag in a sunny spot. The herbs will dry fully within a day or two.

protect yourself while outdoors

Everyone needs to protect themselves from lawn-moving accidents, which are surprisingly common. But people with diabetes also need to make a special effort to protect their feet from blisters and injury, their skin from sunburn, and their bodies from dehydration. Here's how to stay safe while getting exercise outdoors.

Wear breathable cotton trousers and long-sleeved shirts. Anyone who does yard work with bare arms or legs knows how easy it is to pick up scrapes, scratches, and insect bites. They're all injuries you might not have noticed otherwise, but they can get infected in no time. Avoid very loose clothing that could get caught in machinery.

Always wear work gloves. Even moderate yard work will take a toll on your hands. Apart from scratches and nicks here and there, you're bound

Outdoor Projects: Exercise Your Options

Once a month, keep your body moving with one of these "yard upgrade" projects. To keep yourself on task, flip open your calendar and schedule these and other tasks months in advance—you'll be more likely to accomplish the tasks if you write them down.

Install a stone border. Pull up the rubber barrier that delineates the border of your flower garden and install in its place a handsome stone border. Your home store offers a variety of options in prefabricated stone.

Install stepping-stones. Lay stepping-stones in your backyard, flush to the ground, following the most commonly traveled route from your back door to the side yard.

Reorganize your shed. Empty your shed and lay all of your tools and items on the lawn. Throw out everything that's broken or is no longer needed. Cluster like objects together (garden tools, leaf rakes,

car-washing gear, etc.). If necessary, install extra hooks and shelving in the shed to accommodate these tools.

Rearrange the "furniture." Devise a new look for your yard by establishing new positions for your lawn chairs, bench, picnic table, birdbath, and planters. If you're great at plotting it all out in your head, fine. Otherwise sketch your plan on graph paper. It'll look like you have a new yard.

Reseal the deck. Depending on what your deck is made of and what kind of sealer you use, you may need to reseal it every one or two years to protect the wood from deterioration.

Reseal your asphalt driveway. Experts disagree on how much protection driveway sealant provides. But two things are inarguable: A new coating gives your house nice "curb appeal," and it also provides a full afternoon's workout.

golden rule! Always Wear Shoes

Did you know that the spray from a power washer is powerful enough to cut through your toes? Without exception, you should always wear sturdy shoes—those with good support and rubber soles—any time you're in the yard to prevent falls and foot injuries. Bare feet, sandals, and flip-flops are out of the question. Even in a well-kept lawn, there are just too many opportunities to step on sharp objects. Further protect your feet by wearing the right socks. If the nerves in your feet are damaged, the odds that a blister will develop and get infected are high because you may not be able to feel the blister developing. Look for socks that are seamless, have a padded sole, fit snugly without restricting your blood flow, and don't bunch up. Instead of cotton, choose man-made materials that wick moisture away from the skin.

to get a few blisters. Buy multiple sets of work gloves and stash them wherever your other tools and materials for yard work are stored. If you're going to handle anything sharp—for instance, if you're changing the blade on your lawnmower—use heavy-duty gloves with thick leather or Kevlar to protect your palms.

Before you get going on yard work, play pickup sticks (and stones and glass). Before you start trimming hedges, pulling weeds, and mowing the lawn, grab a bucket and stroll around the property for 10 minutes. Toss into the bucket any yard debris that could cause injury while you work, including glass, stones, wire, sticks, nails, and misplaced toys. All of these items become missiles if they're thrown by a power tool.

Take action to prevent lawn-mowing accidents. If you have a push mower, mow across the face of any slopes instead of up and down the hill, and don't pull the mower backward. This will reduce the risk of slipping and being injured by the machine. If you have a riding mower, drive it up and down gradual slopes and avoid steep slopes altogether. Mow only in daylight, and make sure you can see at least four feet in front of the mower. If your mower is self-propelled, never stand in front of it, and always disengage the drive clutch when you start it.

Rub on plenty of sunblock 30 minutes before heading outside. Use sunscreen even on cloudy days. Choose one with an SPF of at least 25. A sunscreen that contains moisturizer is especially useful. When your skin is shielded from damaging sun and kept moist, it's less likely to blister or crack—an invitation to infection.

Get yard work in before 10 a.m. or after 4 p.m. A study conducted by researchers at Loma Linda University and Azusa Pacific University, both in California, shows that people who have diabetes have low tolerance for heat because they seem to sweat less than people who don't have diabetes. Because of the effect that heat has on your body, it's particularly important not to spend extended periods of time outdoors between 10 a.m. and 4 p.m., when the sun's rays are strongest. Scheduling your "yard time" early or in the late afternoon can help you maintain a healthy body temperature.

Drink extra water while working outside. To stay well hydrated, most people need a minimum of eight to 10 8-ounce glasses of water a day; when you're working outdoors in the heat, you should drink even more. Before you head for the yard, take a sports jug—one that holds at least 2 quarts of water—and fill it with ice water. Park the jug in a prominent place in the yard so you'll remember to take a swig every 15 minutes or so. This will prevent dehydration, which can send blood sugar soaring. And water keeps you from feeling hungry.

chapter six

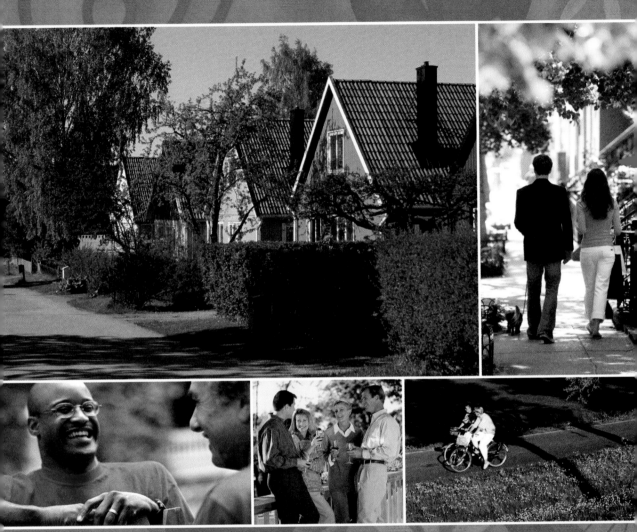

in your neighborhood

You may see your neighborhood as a mere collection of houses,
but it's so much more—there are walking paths right outside
your door, friends to be made, and nearby resources to lean on.
Make the most of it!

step out in the 'hood

You don't have to climb Mount Everest to get fit; you can do it right in your own neighborhood. Recent research shows that getting 30 minutes a day of any type of moderate physical activity can be as powerful as the best diabetes medications available. Exercise boosts not only your energy and your mood, but also your cells' sensitivity to insulin, which allows your cells to soak up more glucose and lowers blood sugar levels. Get moving with these simple strategies.

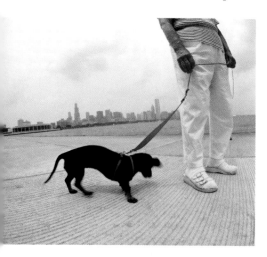

Walk Fido every day. Dog owners walk more than people without dogs. Not surprisingly, they also tend to be healthier, with less body fat, according to a new study from the University of California, San Diego. But not every pooch "parent" takes advantage of these exercise opportunities. And those who don't walk their four-legged friends don't get the health perks. If you don't own a dog, offer to take the neighbor's dog for a walk, or join your neighbor in his or her daily jaunt.

Volunteer at a local animal shelter to walk a pooch several times a week. Most shelters will let you participate with a little bit of training. Have a favorite breed? You can find rescue centers for labs, retrievers, even Schnoodles (Schnauzer/poodle mixes) by asking at your local humane society, animal shelter, or veterinary hospital. You can also try searching online by typing in the name of the breed, "rescue center," and your town.

Sweep and weed your sidewalk once a week. Making a habit of keeping a tidy path in front of your house will make it more inviting to others, give you a chance to say hello to your fellow citizens while you're weeding—and burn off 100 calories in just 20 minutes of vigorous work.

Stroll to your neighborhood mailbox. Instead of leaving outgoing mail in your home mailbox, walk your bill, magazine subscription, or birthday card to the government mailbox a few blocks away, or even to the post office if it's within a mile or so from your home. Not only will you benefit from the blood-sugar-stabilizing activity, your check will be safer than it would be sitting in front of your house.

Return misdelivered mail to its rightful home on foot. It happens to everyone: You get a letter that should have gone to the house one or two blocks over. Instead of marking it "wrong address" and clipping it to your mailbox, look at the post as an opportunity to get a few minutes of activity, some fresh air, and a chance to meet a neighbor.

Take your newspaper on a daily walk. When you step outside for your morning paper, take the opportunity to go around your block one time. The fresh morning air will help wake you up—sans caffeine—and you'll start your day off right with a few extra steps. You'll knock off five minutes of exercise from your 30-minutes-a-day goal before you even sit down to have breakfast.

Take advantage of your sidewalk. It's there, it's free, and all you need is a good pair of walking shoes to use it. Begin gradually, with a 15- to 20-minute walk. Start strolling slowly for about three to five minutes, then pick up your pace for 10 minutes and cool down for another three to five minutes. Each week, add two to three minutes to the faster portion of your walk. Within a few weeks, you'll be up to walking briskly for 30 minutes most days a week.

Try out a pair of walking poles. You'll burn far more calories on your neighborhood walks with these poles, which you use like a cross-country skier. Called fitness trekking or Nordic walking, walking with these poles can boost your calorie burn 20 to 50 percent over regular strolling because the poles recruit the muscles in your upper body. Poles can also be helpful if you need a little extra stability or want to take some impact off of your legs. Follow the instructions that come with the poles. You might also be able to find a lesson through your local health club, community center, or YMCA. You can order poles and get instructional tips at www.exerstrider.com or www.nordicwalking.com.

Say your ABCs out loud. When you're out walking for exercise, your pace shouldn't be so tough that you're gasping for air, or so easy that you can babble nonstop to your exercise buddy without breaking a sweat. If you're by yourself, recite the alphabet. If it's no problem, pick up your pace. If you start huffing by the letter F, slow down.

Rate your exercise intensity. Another good rule of thumb: On a scale of 1 to 10, 10 being running as fast as you can, and 1 being sitting on the couch, you want to aim for about a 6 or 7. At that intensity, you should be breathing harder than normal but still able to carry on a simple conversation.

Clip on a pedometer in the morning. The little gadget will keep track of how many steps you take that day—and subtly encourage you to take even more. Try to take 500 additional steps each week, aiming

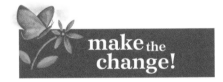

make the change!

The habit: Walking 30 minutes a day.

The result: You'll live longer.

The proof: Walking just over eight blocks a day can slash your risk of premature death by more than a third. Go a little farther, and you'll cut your risk by up to 50 percent, according to a study from the Centers for Disease Control and Prevention. After comparing activity levels and death rates of almost 2,900 adults with diabetes over the course of 11 years, researchers found that walkers lived longer than those who were sedentary.

ultimately for as many as 10,000 steps a day. In case you're curious, 1,000 steps equal one-half mile.

Keep a step log. It takes approximately six months for a new behavior to become habit. To help you lock in your walking habit, write down your steps after you take off your pedometer every night. Recording your progress helps you stay focused.

Crummy weather? Take a mall walk. Check your mall to see if they offer a mall-walking program or early morning hours for walkers. If it doesn't, you can still get there first thing in the morning—hours before the teens get out of bed—do a few laps, and then treat yourself to a skim milk latte. Invite a friend along, and agree to do one quick lap for some harder exercise, and then one moderate lap for a little bit of window shopping—then repeat, one fast lap/one relaxed, on the upper level.

Promote your own mall-walking program. If your mall doesn't have a walking program, consider talking to the mall management. Some malls don't want to be responsible for possible injuries, and if this is the case, suggest that the staff develop a consent form that walkers must sign before joining the program. If you have friends, neighbors, and coworkers who want to mall walk, ask them to call the public relations department of the mall to express their interest. You may even want to volunteer your time to get the program under way.

Print up a flyer to advertise for walking buddies. Post them around your block, in your church, or at the local grocery store. Invite folks to meet you on Thursday evenings at six o'clock, or whatever works best for you, and

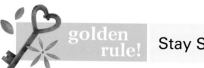

golden rule! Stay Safe on Walks

In case of an emergency it's a good idea to pack a few items when you head outdoors. A fanny pack with zippered pouches and a water holder is perfect (you can find these at sporting good stores). Always bring water and drink it at regular intervals whether you feel thirsty or not; dehydration can make blood sugar skyrocket. Stash some glucose tablets in one of the zippered pouches. It's also wise to bring a cell phone. In many areas it is becoming popular to store an "In Case of Emergency" (ICE) contact number in your phone. Before the person's name, type in ICE in the contact list (for example, ICE Steve). Last but certainly not least, people with diabetes should wear some sort of identification—a medical ID bracelet or necklace or a tag on a watch—stating that they have diabetes and indicating if they are on insulin or another medication that can cause hypoglycemia.

include your first name, number, and e-mail address. Pick a place to meet, such as a park, community center, or nearby library. Remember to start and finish your walk with five minutes of slower strolling to warm up and cool down your muscles.

Formalize your new walking club. Arrange to convene at a local coffee shop following your first or second walk. Hand out name tags and have a sign-in sheet for everyone to list their names, phone numbers, and e-mail addresses so you can contact them about future walks. Next discuss how often you'll walk, when and where to meet, what to do in case of bad weather, the speed of the walk, and the distance you'll cover. If you have a large group, consider breaking into smaller groups based on fitness level, availability, or other factors.

Look for ways to motivate the group. You might choose a name for your walking crew, order shirts, have a monthly potluck (healthy of course), enter a walking event with a cause, or set goals to increase the length of your walks or your walking pace. Share the responsibility by asking each member to lead some of the walks and have them plan the route.

Use your car to clock errands you could do on foot. Put a sticky note on your dashboard that says "Clock a route" to remind you to check the mileage on all the places you typically go in a day. Is the library a mile away? How about the ATM? Many people don't realize how many errands could be done on foot with a little planning, says Mark Fenton, world-renowned environmental walking coach.

Grab binoculars and go bird watching. You can pick up a beginning birding book at a local bookstore. Look for one that includes birds in your region. It's a great way to enjoy nature and connect with wildlife right in your own community. Observing the beauty of birds and discussing them with friends, neighbors, or your children can be a fun and stimulating experience. Interacting with nature tends to slow the heart rate, reduce blood pressure, and help people relax.

Put a "Could I walk or ride my bike?" sticky note on your front door. Having a prompt (like the famous string around the finger) in plain view will cue you to ask yourself if you really need to hop in your car to take the books back to the library, pick up a prescription, or visit a friend. Post a second note on your dash that says "Could I walk halfway?" so you'll be encouraged to park a few blocks from whatever errand you're running.

Go on a village scavenger hunt. Whether you have kids, grandkids, nieces, or nephews, this activity never fails: Jot a list that includes items such as five red cars, three houses with yellow daisies, two cats, four stop

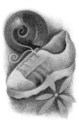

Ask yourself if you really need to hop in the car or if you could go by foot or by bike.

signs, and so on. After you've compiled several "treasures" for the kids to find, head out around the neighborhood until you've found all the items on the list. You can make several lists and have friendly competitions. The first one to complete the list wins.

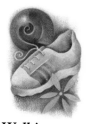

Walking shoes will encourage you to move more and will decrease your risk of injury.

Make after-dinner walks a regular habit. Instead of collapsing in front of the TiVo, create a tradition of post-meal strolls with a partner. If you have young kids, you can play games to keep the little ones entertained. Remember the Alphabet Game during long family car trips? You can play it while walking. Look for signs, bumper stickers, and personalized license plates on cars, and watch for words that begin with each letter of the alphabet. Once you've found one letter, move on to the next.

Make a list of five active things you can do in your community. Hang the list on your fridge, and when you're out of ideas for an active weekend activity, look to your list. For example, you could bike to a local park for a picnic, hoof it to the library, or plan to meet friends at a halfway location to which you can both walk.

Have a monthly trash patrol day. Grab a shopping bag and head out around your block for 20 minutes. Rope in a few neighbors to join you. Every time you have to bend to pick up an article, turn the move into a squat: Extend your buttocks behind you and pretend you're about to sit in an invisible chair until your upper legs are almost parallel to the ground. You'll build leg muscles and sculpt your rear view. Building muscle helps the body become more insulin sensitive, and it boosts your metabolism.

Lace up walking shoes for active living every day. You may think that any old shoe is fine, but footwear designed for walking will encourage you to move more and will decrease your risk of injury. A good shoe should be flexible in the ball of the foot, but not in the arch. (A shoe that bends in the arch can put strain on tendons in the feet.) The heel should be cushioned (because that's where your foot strikes) and also rounded to encourage an easy and speedy heel-toe motion. It's best to visit a local, independently owned running store. Whether you have low or high arches, the salespeople in a competent technical fitness store will watch you walk barefoot and help you choose the features you need.

Burn calories at the little ones' soccer games. Instead of taking your folding chair and a crossword puzzle, wear comfortable shoes and take a jaunt around the field during soccer or baseball games when your child isn't playing. You can still cheer while in motion. Or take your walk before the game starts, when the kids are warming up. Remember, physical activity enhances the action of insulin (the hormone that lowers your blood sugar), which often results in better blood sugar control.

get to know your neighbors

The more social you are, the healthier you're likely to be. People who know others in their community tend to be less stressed and happier than folks who live in isolation. Anxiety can raise stress hormones in your body that can in turn raise blood sugar and exacerbate insulin resistance. So use one of these excuses to get yourself out of the house or invite others over.

Plan an annual block party. Contact your local police department for information about permits and make flyers well ahead of time to round up a group of block party committee leaders. Be sure to plan healthy activities such as scavenger hunts, hide and seek, and flag football. Make a menu sign-up list that has plenty of healthy vegetable dishes and fresh fruit options—and don't forget lots of bottled water so you stay hydrated and don't waste precious calories on soda or alcohol.

Have a weekly comedy night with the neighbors. Gather the gals or guys on your street to watch a weekly TV show you all love and can laugh at together. Not only does laughing increase those feel-good hormones called endorphins, it also decreases blood pressure, pain, anxiety—and even blood sugar! A study from Japan showed that people who watched a comedy show after eating had lower glucose levels than those who didn't. If there's nothing funny on television, take turns sharing your favorite funny movies with friends. If you're going to have food, save it for after the show so you don't unconsciously gobble up too many calories, and suggest that snacks be limited to air-popped popcorn and fresh fruit.

Start a monthly book club. Network with your friends and neighbors to find interested members, or visit your local library, church, community

---

whip it together!   Picnic Lemon Rice Salad

Bring something a little different this year to the gang. A cool rice salad is just perfect for those hot days. Easy to tote and with a fresh lemon taste, it's a light dish that goes with any grilled seafood or poultry.

Combine 2 cups cooked **brown rice** with 1 cup diced seeded **tomato**, 1 cup thawed **frozen green peas**, 1 peeled and diced **carrot**, 2 minced **scallions**, and ¼ cup minced fresh **parsley**. Whisk together 3 tablespoons of nonfat **mayonnaise**, 1 tablespoon of **lemon juice**, ½ teaspoon of **lemon zest**, and **salt** and **pepper** to taste. Add to the rice salad and toss well.

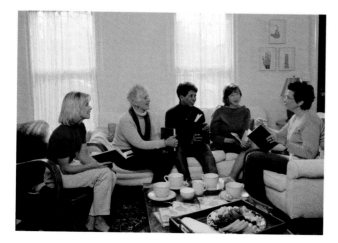

center, or independent bookstore to post flyers inviting people to e-mail or call in their interest. You can either have round-robin meetings where each meeting is held at a different person's house, or ask if one of the establishments above would be willing to host meetings.

Too busy to read books? No worry: Buy or rent audio books. Listen to them on your walks, then get together with the group to discuss.

Attend a monthly neighborhood council meeting. You'll stay apprised of the happenings, find volunteering opportunities, and meet others in your community. Call your city or check the local section of your newspaper to find out when and where meetings are held. If you get involved, you might have a chance to promote some of the walking ideas mentioned earlier.

Log on to www.diabetes.org to find local events. This is the Web site of the American Diabetes Association. Click on the Community, Workplace, and Local Events tab on its home page to find information on diabetes walks or investigate how to promote your own local support groups.

Organize a local bike ride, or get involved with Tour de Cure, a series of cycling events held in more than 80 cities nationwide to benefit the American Diabetes Association. The Tour is a ride, not a race, with routes designed for everyone from the occasional rider to the experienced cyclist. Regardless of your experience level, you'll travel a route supported from start to finish with rest stops, food to replenish your energy, and fans and volunteers cheering you on. Find more information about Tour de Cure at www.diabetes.org.

Visit your elders once a month. It's as simple as pulling out your yellow pages and calling nearby assisted living facilities. There are also organizations that deliver meals to seniors, and you can volunteer for those as well. Look for resources in your community at www.mealcall.org. Another option is to check with your place of worship. You can visit someone who is in the hospital for a short stay or adjusting to a new apartment. Not sure what to talk about? People love to talk about themselves. Ask historical questions. Not sure what to do? Bring flowers, a book to share, a checkerboard, some dominoes, or a deck of cards.

socialize the healthy way

Unfortunately, get-togethers can often have their own stressors thanks to the abundance of bad-for-you foods. For strategies on protecting your blood sugar levels without sacrificing your social circle, read on.

Eyeball the offerings at church socials *before* you start to fill your plate. It's all too easy to load up a volcano-size pile of mashed potatoes, maca-roni salad, lasagna, chips, and brownies if you just hop in line and start piling things on your plate. But if you take a minute to examine all the offerings first, you'll make better choices. Pass up the fried chicken and look for healthier items with which to fill your plate.

Bring a healthy dish to barbecues and picnics. That will ensure there's at least one thing you can scoop up without straying from your eating plan. Try bringing a fruit salad, a tomato and cucumber salad, a juicy watermel-on, or a platter of fresh veggies and low-fat ranch dressing or hummus. For the grill, offer chicken kabobs with onions, mushrooms, and cherry toma-toes interspersed with the chicken.

Keep your hands busy at summer picnics and events. Stay away from plentiful temptations such as chips and sweets by offering to be the official event photographer or starting a game of horseshoes or volleyball.

Have only one glass of wine or one beer. If you can keep your alcohol consumption to one drink or under, you're probably okay, since most stud-ies don't show increased risks for a single glass. Skip mixed cocktails, since they tend to be loaded with sugar, calories, and carbs, and don't drink on an empty stomach because it can spike blood sugar.

whip it together! | Mexicali Corn, Chicken, and Bean Pot Luck

You might just have to plan on preparing a double batch of this simple, fiber-rich, one-pot dish after it all disappears at your next neighborhood get-together. It can be prepared a day in advance.

In a large bowl, mix together 1 diced **red bell pepper**, 2 sliced **scallions**, 1 can (15-ounces) drained and rinsed **black beans**, 1 package (10 ounces) thawed **frozen corn kernels**, and 6 ounces diced cooked **white meat chicken**. Whisk together 2½ tablespoons **olive oil**, 1½ tablespoons fresh **lime juice**, 1 tablespoon **red wine vinegar**, 2 minced **garlic** cloves, ½ teaspoon **chili powder**, and **salt** and **pepper** to taste. Add the dressing to the bean and corn mixture and toss well.

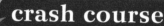

how to start a community garden

The very freshest fruits and vegetables come straight from the ground, and a fun and inexpensive way to get more of them is to start a community garden. Besides the good that comes from giving back to your community, you'll gain the health benefits that come from socializing and from the gardening itself—digging, weeding, watering, hoeing, raking—which burns plenty of calories and builds muscle to keep you slim and lower your blood sugar. Here is a guide to help you get started.

1 | recruit help

Enlist two or three area residents or friends to join you. This will help take some of the workload of starting up the garden off your shoulders. You can also connect with people through neighborhood associations, gardening clubs, your church, or a civic association. Most people will not travel far to garden, so put your recruiting efforts into a two-mile radius of the possible garden location. Another idea is to get involved with a school district. Many encourage gardens as part of an educational program, and they are always looking for volunteers who'd like to get involved and teach the next generation about gardening. The National Gardening Association (www.gardening.org) has information about starting a school-based garden in your area.

2 | find a plot

The biggest issue is finding the land to use. You'll need a site that gets at least six hours of full sunlight daily and has access to water.

Start by seeing what resources exist in your neighborhood. If you have an area in mind, such as an empty lot near your house, ask at the neighboring houses or businesses about who owns the property, contact them, and see

if they'd be interested in sponsoring a neighborhood garden. "Many cities offer yearlong leases for $1 on vacant properties, so check with your local city department," says Lexie Stoia, operations administrator for the American Community Gardening Association. Note that you may need to buy liability insurance. Also check with your parks and recreation department; it's possible you might be able to use park land.

Before you invest your time, check that a community garden doesn't already exist in your area. Ask around, search online for "community garden" and the name of your town, or log onto www.communitygarden.org, which also offers plenty of information and tips.

Before you commit to any land, do a soil check. You can find a soil test lab by searching online or by asking at a local nursery, agriculture college, or cooperative extension office. Finally, be sure to check with your city hall or police station about required permits.

3 | get to know your region

If you're an experienced gardener, chances are you already know what you want to plant and when to plant it. But if you are new to gardening, you'll want to do some homework or get

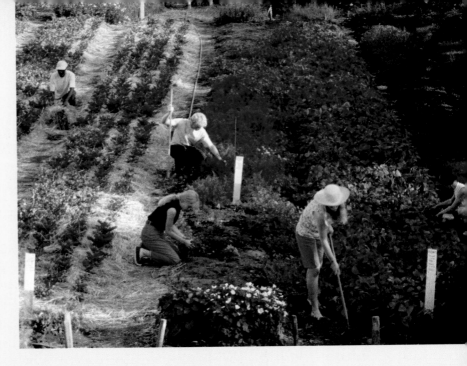

an experienced part-
ner. Beginning
gardening books can
tell you what typically
grows in each season,
how often you'll need
to water and fertilize,
how to prepare the
soil, how to sketch a
garden plot with what
is to be planted where,
and what tools you'll
need. For information
on gardening in your
region, contact your
local cooperative
extension office. They can provide you with
free information about horticulture, pest control, and soil for your area. Check out
www.csrees.usda.gov/Extension to find the
office nearest you.

4 | create a garden committee

The size and experience level of the group
you'll need will depend on the size of land you
have to plant and how complex you'd like the
garden to be. Maybe you will need only a few
friends, or maybe you're looking to have a large
neighborhood resource. Decide on a meeting
place and time (ask your community center,
library, or coffee shop if they would host a
meeting), then post flyers at the local gardening club, school district, library, community
center, coffee shops, bookstores, post office,
and the local college's agriculture department,
if there is one.

5 | have a kickoff meeting

At the first meeting, you can decide on issues
such as what vegetables to plant, whether you
want to have individual plots or one coopera-
tively managed garden, and how you'll get

funds to start gardening. Maybe each person
can bring their own gardening tools each time
you meet, but you'll still need to decide on
how you'll want to get seeds or small plants.
Does the group want to seek funding and
donations to work on the property, or would
the group prefer to pay membership dues that
would cover the costs of seeds, tools, fertilizer,
and other needed items? You should also
decided on how you'll rotate your weekly
weeding, watering, and pruning schedule
among members. Finally, decide on a meeting
schedule, starting with a beginning date for
preparing the gardening plot.

6 | prepare your plot

Most of your first work day will be spent
preparing the soil. You'll need to clean the site
of any weeds, turn or plow the soil, and fertilize. You can also use the first day to formalize
your garden plan and decide on plot sizes and
responsibilities for various sections. Be sure to
include a compost area so you can create your
own garden fertilizer from plant leftovers.
After the soil is ready, meet for your first
planting day.

lean on community resources

There are multitudes of community-based opportunities for improving your overall health, your fitness, and your diet. Open your eyes and look around to see where those opportunities are. Here are a few tips to get you started.

Join a public pool or a local YMCA. For a minimal membership fee, most Ys or health clubs will allow you access to their pools so you can swim laps or take a water aerobics class. There's no kinder, gentler place to start working out than in gravity-defying water. Swimming is easy on your joints, burns tons of calories, and makes you feel like a kid on summer vacation, all while giving you grown-up fitness and muscle tone. Since you weigh only 10 to 15 percent of your land weight in the water, swimming or water exercise classes are great for people who have nerve damage that affects their feet and who need to avoid too much weight-bearing activity.

Sign up for group strength-training classes at a local gym or through a continuing education program. Resistance (weight) training is just as important as aerobic exercise for diabetes control. In fact, it's better than aerobic exercises at increasing insulin sensitivity, lowering your risk for thinning bones, and preventing loss of muscle that slows metabolism. Group classes can be more fun, and safer, then using strength machines.

Get personal with your own trainer. Another way to tap into strength training is to find a certified personal trainer who has a local studio, works in your health club, or will come to your home. Many trainers offer family, pair, or small-group training at more affordable prices. Having weekly sessions for a month or two is a great way to learn an individualized program that starts at your level and meets your personal strength needs. You can search for a personal trainer in your area by asking at your local gym or searching online at www.acefitness.org.

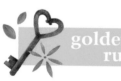

golden rule! Don't Let Two Days Go By Without Exercising

Experts know that going without physical activity makes the body use insulin less efficiently, which in turn makes blood sugar harder to control. Now researchers at the University of Missouri at Columbia studying lab animals have shown that when rats weren't allowed to run on their exercise wheels for two days, the amount of sugar taken into their muscle cells in response to insulin was cut by about a third. Whether or not the exact results apply to humans, the advice is the same: Unless you're sick, move your body every day.

Take a healthy cooking class. Look for courses through local community colleges or high school continuing education programs. Go for general healthy cooking or get creative and sign up for a vegetarian, Mediterranean, or Asian cooking class. It's a fun, productive way to get out of the house.

Visit a local meal-assembly store to get "homemade" meals in a hurry. Companies that let you assemble your own meals from fresh or frozen ingredients already laid out for you are cropping up all over the country. Just sign up, show up, choose your menus, then rotate through different workstations to assemble your meals in containers they provide. Take them home in a cooler, decide what's for dinner, and put the rest in the freezer. Thawing and heating instructions are provided. No grocery trips, no cleanup! Invite friends and make it a social outing. Try searching online under meal assembly and your city, look in your newspaper's food section, or search through the vendors listed on www.easymealprep.com to see if there's one in your area.

Treat yourself to weekly trips to the farmers' market. You'll find the freshest fruits and vegetables there, and some interesting varieties you won't find at the grocery store. Plus, the produce tends to be local and organic— good for the environment and your health. You may even meet other locals who are invested in community and good health. Look in your local paper, call your city hall, or visit www.localharvest.org to search for markets near you.

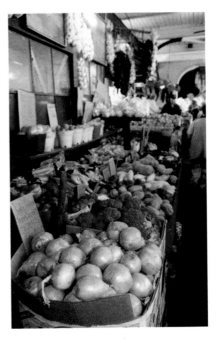

Sign up for a yoga class at a local center or YMCA. It's another great way to lower stress. According to one recent study from California State University in San Bernardino, adults reported significant decreases in anxiety and increases in motivation and concentration after just eight weeks of practicing a relaxing form of yoga, compared to a control group. To start, choose a gentle form of yoga such as Hatha that includes relaxing breathing.

Head for a place of worship. Following their faith helps many people put stressors in place by reminding them of what really matters in life. Attending a local church or temple also provides a sanctuary from life's stresses that you can enjoy with others who share your beliefs. The same community can help you out during tough times.

volunteer to get out of the house

One of the best ways to improve your health is to help others. Whether it's at your place of worship, library, or humane society, volunteering makes you feel good and gets you out of the house more often, increasing your activity level and improving your self-esteem. Helping others can lower your risk of depression, high blood pressure, and heart disease. You'll even live longer, according to a recent report from the Corporation for National and Community Services, based in Washington, DC.

Do chores for an ailing neighbor. Combine the obvious health benefits of exercise and fresh air with subtler feel-good benefits that come from doing good deeds. Offer to mow the lawn, shovel the driveway, water the plants, or walk the dog. Or bring by some library books, a few rented DVDs, or a home-baked meal for your homebound neighbor.

If you have kids, start a walking school bus. It's like a carpool—without the car—and with the added benefits of exercise and socializing with friends and neighbors. This can be as informal as two neighboring families taking turns walking their children to school, or as structured as a route with several meeting points, a timetable, and a regularly rotated schedule. To get started, invite families who live nearby to walk, pick a route to your child's school and take a test walk, and decide how often the group will walk together (you can start with one, two, or three days a week). Visit www.walkingschoolbus.org for more information.

Volunteer to coach or referee for a community soccer, basketball, or football team—or umpire a Little League baseball game. Alternatively, you could volunteer to help run drills or do jumping jacks with kids during their warm-up time. Coaches of young kids' teams often appreciate an extra hand.

Read to others. Even if your children are grown, your community is full of kids who need volunteer grandparents, aunts, and uncles to read at local schools or day-care centers. What better way to pass on your wisdom to the next generation? If you offer to volunteer at a school or child-care facility, be prepared to fill out some forms and have a health check. Alternatively, you could help an illiterate adult learn to read. Many libraries have volunteer programs and offer free training on helping adults learn to read.

chapter seven

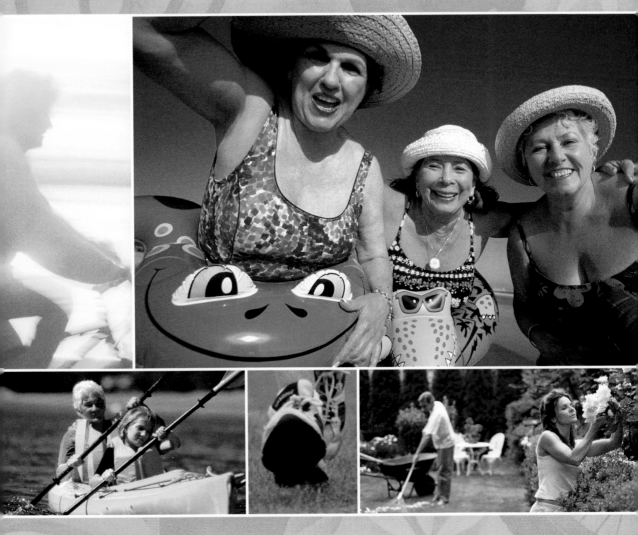

on your playground

As children, we ran ourselves ragged in the yard, in the pool, on the ball field, and wherever else we could find to play. We didn't think of it as "exercise" then, so why start now? Get out of the house and have some fun!

keep it fun

You don't have to be one of those 10-mile-a-day runners or a Tour de France cyclist to be an active person. Focus on sports and hobbies you love. Do them often, and you'll find yourself in better shape—and maybe even a happier person—in no time. And it won't even seem like effort.

Don't fret about aerobic versus strength training. Experts conclude that aerobic activity (walking and cycling, for instance) and strength training (lifting weights and doing strength exercises) are almost equally beneficial for controlling blood sugar, so pick whichever most appeals to you. Aerobic activity causes your muscles to burn energy and then draw glucose out of the blood to replace that energy, thus lowering your blood sugar. Strength training gives your body a larger mass of muscle, so there are more cells drawing glucose out of your bloodstream at any one time—another path to lower blood sugar.

Sign up for something fun. You might be turned off by the prospect of huffing your way around a running track or grunting your way through a series of weight machines at the gym, so appeal instead to the human desire for fun. Try a swimming-pool aerobics class that plays oldies music, sign up for tango lessons and dress the part, join a hiking club to become one with nature, or volunteer to give walking tours at an arboretum.

Invest in professional lessons, classes, or retreats. You may do a double take when you find out the price of a three-day yoga retreat, but if you're going to splurge on something, your health should be at the top of the list. When you pay an expert to show you how to use weight machines properly, to ride a horse, or belly dance, you'll master the skill faster and enjoy your pursuit more. And a lesson is a small price to pay to keep from injuring yourself.

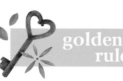

golden rule!   Choose an Activity That Makes You Feel Alive

People who play tennis every week, take a daily swim in the ocean, or hit the golf links whenever there's an open tee time don't do it for the exercise; they do it because they love it. (That doesn't mean it doesn't sometimes frustrate them to the point of throwing tennis rackets or golf clubs!) You may not love a new sport in the beginning, when your skills aren't quite up to snuff, so give it some time. But do choose a sport or activity you're naturally drawn to—that you simply think is fun or emotionally satisfying—and you'll be much more likely to stick with it and not view it as exercise.

Try yoga or tai chi class. You don't have to work up a sweat to get a benefit—or three—from exercise. Both yoga and tai chi increase your flexibility and balance. The slow, sure movements and gentle stretching not only benefit your muscles and joints but also your mental health—their stress-relief benefits are proven. Since being stressed can raise your blood pressure and drive your blood sugar down, or more often, up, those 45 minutes in class can do you more good than you realize.

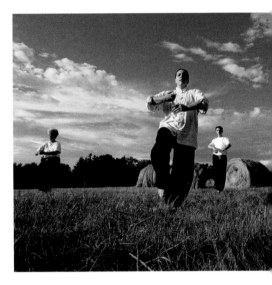

If you love people, keep it social. If you've got the gift of gab or are always up for meeting new friends, seek out group activities such as volleyball, shuffleboard, bocce, and bowling. Staying socially connected is a key to keeping your spirits up. And you know what they say: Laughter is the best medicine. If you have a good time with the people you're exercising with, chances are you'll keep coming back for more.

Hang around fun, active people. If you have friends who love to hike or hit the driving range, their enthusiasm is likely to rub off on you. And most sports are more fun when you play them with friends. A study at the University of Iceland found that men whose fathers, brothers, and close friends exercised with them (or who emphasized exercise in their own lives) were more likely to exercise and be fit than those whose friends and family did not participate.

Vary your activities. Your passion for racquetball is bound to wane if you keep doing it day in and day out. Give yourself a break from your favorite game and go country line dancing or hiking in the great outdoors once in a while for a change of pace. If mountain biking is your thing, trade in your spokes for some strokes at the swimming pool.

Train for an event. Whether it's a 5-mile "fun run" or a walk for a good cause, put it on your calendar, then get out there and get ready. Give yourself plenty of time to work up gradually to the amount of walking or running you'll be doing.

Have a passion for helping? Volunteer to use your muscle. That is, offer to do manual labor for an organization that helps less-fortunate people. For instance, Habitat for Humanity International will put you to work painting, nailing, and hauling materials as you build homes for the poor. Not only will your body benefit, but your spirit will, too, knowing the good you have done.

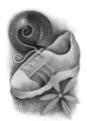

You should not feel pain or shortness of breath while exercising.

exercise smarts

There's little or no excuse for people with diabetes to skip exercise because of their "condition." The fact is, people with the disease have scaled mountains, trekked across nations, won professional tennis matches, and more. That said, it does pay to play it smart when you're exercising. Start by following these tips.

If you have trouble standing, sit and exercise. Don't let limited use of your legs or unsteadiness on your feet stop you from getting fit. Buy an exercise video designed for people sitting in a wheelchair or chair. A good one will give you a heart-healthy aerobic workout and build your upper-body muscles as well. Such videos work well for people who are new to physical activity, even if they have full use of their legs. Many people are surprised to discover that they can work up a good sweat while sitting down. To get maximum enjoyment out of your sessions, find a video with an engaging host and upbeat music that will keep you moving.

Go easy on yourself if you're under the weather. If you've got the sniffles or have come down with the mystery "bug" that's going around, exercise only if you feel like you have the energy and stamina to do so. If you don't feel up to it, give your body the rest it needs, and resume your regular exercise routine when you feel better.

Ease up if you're struggling. If you find yourself breathing heavily or you otherwise feel uncomfortable, you might be overexerting yourself. It's time to ease up. Give yourself the "talk test": Speak one complete sentence aloud. If you have trouble doing it, slow your pace. You should not feel pain, extreme fatigue, or shortness of breath.

To speed your walking pace, take more strides, not longer ones. When you challenge yourself by quickening the pace of your walking or running,

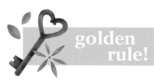

golden rule!   ## Listen to Your Body

Because people with diabetes are at such a high risk of cardiovascular disease, it's important to tune in to what your body is telling you while you exercise. Stop exercising immediately if you experience chest, arm, or jaw pain; nausea, dizziness, or fainting (which are also signs of heat exhaustion or hypoglycemia); unusual shortness of breath; or an irregular heart beat. All are signs of heart problems and should be checked out right away. For people with diabetes, the mantra "No pain, no gain" definitely does not apply.

move faster by increasing the number of steps you take in a given time—not by increasing the length of your stride. It's more efficient, and if you lengthen your stride, the motion could injure your feet, knees, or shins.

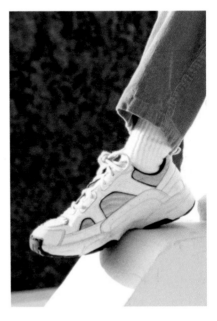

Buy athletic shoes that feel comfortable the first time you try them on. Don't tell yourself that your sneakers will feel better when they're broken in. Ill-fitting shoes can rub your feet raw, which could lead to a dangerous infection. Whether you're buying shoes for tennis, walking, bowling, or any other sport, choose the highest-quality shoe you can afford, and look for a model with ventilation that will allow the shoe to "breathe." If you have reduced feeling in your feet due to nerve damage, you may need a podiatrist or a shoe-fitting expert to find the right sneaker for you.

Wear soft, sweat-wicking athletic socks. Before you work out, pull on a clean pair of cushiony athletic socks. Socks made from a cotton-and-synthetic blend are ideal because they wick moisture away from your feet. If your feet get moist, your skin will blister more easily.

Make sure your insulin pump's infusion set will stay put. If you wear an insulin pump while you're physically active, apply antiperspirant or liquid bandage adhesive (such as Mastisol) to the skin around your insulin pump's infusion set before taping it. This will help prevent sweat from loosening the infusion set's adhesive from your skin. Cover the infusion site with a small cotton ball, spray the antiperspirant on the surrounding skin, and allow it to dry before you exercise. The liquid bandage adhesive is available from online medical supply companies or from insulin pump companies.

Get your "frozen shoulder" to a doctor. For unknown reasons, people with diabetes are particularly prone to a condition called "frozen shoulder." To test the mobility in your shoulder, try this: Lie on your back on the floor with your arms at your sides. Raise your arm in an arc, as if you were doing the backstroke, and try to touch the floor behind your head. If you can come within a few inches of the floor, your range of motion is normal. If not, call your doctor. Early treatment increases your odds of regaining full use of your shoulder.

exercising safely with diabetes

Having diabetes doesn't mean you have to avoid physical activity. It just means that you need to take more precautions than others do when you work out. Here's how to get on the road to regular physical activity and stay the healthy course.

1 | talk to your doctor

Tell your doctor if you're planning to change your activity level. If you're starting an exercise program, the American Diabetes Association recommends a physical exam (and usually a graded exercise test) if you have had type 1 diabetes for more than 15 years, if you have had type 2 diabetes for more than 10 years, if you're sedentary, or if you're over age 35. Your doctor also will want to consider your physical condition—including such issues as heart disease, kidney disease, nerve damage, and eye damage—in helping you decide what kinds of exercise are good fits for you.

Discuss medication changes. Regular physical activity can lessen the amount of insulin or other diabetes medication that you require.

2 | learn when to test and when to rest

If you're on insulin, check your blood sugar before, during, and after exercise. This is the best way to tell how your workout has affected your glucose levels.

Check your blood sugar before exercising if you have type 2 diabetes and you're taking insulin or drugs that prompt the pancreas to produce more insulin. If your glucose is below 100, have a snack that contains carbohydrate before exercising. During a prolonged activity check every 30 minutes to make sure your glucose stays in your target range.

If you're prone to hypoglycemia, check your glucose over the course of several hours after exercise. This applies particularly to people who have type 1 diabetes. Your muscles will continue to pull glucose out of your bloodstream, so taking a reading right after a workout won't give you the full picture of your activity's effect on your glucose levels. You might think your blood sugar is normal while it's actually plummeting. Also, physical activity can speed up how fast insulin goes to work.

Schedule workouts so they follow meals. If you find that you often have to compensate for hypoglycemia by eating a snack during physical activity, see if you do better exercising an hour or two after a meal.

As sport seasons change, adjust food and medications accordingly. For instance, when your recreational tennis league starts up its season, you might be surprised to find your blood sugar running low if you don't account for the twice-a-week tennis practices.

3 | be prepared

Keep essentials with you. If you're working up a sweat away from home, carry a high-carbohydrate snack, diabetes ID (bracelet, necklace, or sneaker tag), and a cell phone for emergencies.

Brief a buddy on emergency procedures. Make sure someone in the vicinity knows that you have diabetes and knows what to do in an emergency. If you're working out at home, make sure a family member is nearby; if you're at the gym, alert a staff member.

Don shoes designed specifically for your sport. That means running shoes for running, soccer shoes for soccer, tennis shoes for tennis, and so on. Sneakers with air or gel cushioning are a good bet because they will absorb shocks to your feet and knees.

Drink plenty of water before exercising. In the two hours before you start working out, drink at least two cups of water.

4 | learn how to warm up and cool down

Start moving around and stretching 5 or 10 minutes before real physical activity. A warm-up can entail a light-and-easy version of the primary exercise. For instance, if you plan to go running, warm up with a 5- or 10-minute walk and then some gentle stretches to get your muscles ready for more intense activity. Weightlifting while your muscles are cold can injure you, too; before you lift anything heavy, raise your body temperature by jogging, riding a stationary bike, or walking on a treadmill.

Cool down gradually. As with the warm-up, do a brief, light version of your workout, keeping your arms and legs moving while your heart rate and breathing slow down.

5 | exercise care while exerting yourself

Exhale during every lift. When you are lifting weights, exhale during exertion and inhale while you are returning the weight to its starting position. Holding your breath while lifting weights can be dangerous. Not only does it raise your blood pressure, but it also raises the pressure within your eyes and can worsen eye diseases to which people with diabetes are vulnerable, such as glaucoma and diabetic retinopathy.

Calories Burned Per 30 Minutes	
Bicycling	272
Cross-country skiing	255
Gardening	170
Golfing (walking with clubs)	187
Hiking	204
Ice skating/roller skating	204
Kayaking/canoeing	170
Racquetball	238
Snowshoeing	272
Swimming	272
Tennis	238
Volleyball (casual)	102

Burn rates are for a person who weighs 150 pounds. Lighter people will burn fewer calories; heavier people will burn more.

Watch for symptoms of hypoglycemia. It's easy to mistake symptoms of hypoglycemia for the effects of exercise. Among the signs of low blood sugar are profuse sweating, rapid heartbeat, trembling, extreme hunger, difficulty thinking, blurred vision, loss of coordination, and "just not feeling right." If you suspect you have hypoglycemia, stop exercising immediately and consume a source of glucose, such as raisins, hard candy, water with fruit juice added to it, or glucose tablets.

If you feel pain, stop exercising. We've said it before, but it is worth repeating: If you start to feel uncomfortable or short of breath when you are exercising, immediately reduce your degree of exertion or stop exercising altogether.

Drink water while you're working out. Experts recommend at least one-half to 1 cup of water every 15 minutes.

Avoid exercising in extreme temperatures. If it's particularly hot or cold outside, find an indoor venue for your workout. In particular, be wary of hot, humid weather because it will be difficult for your body to cool down.

on the court or course

Ask a golfer walking the fairgrounds what he's doing. Chances are he won't say "exercising." Same goes for someone trying to perfect her tennis serve. Sports like tennis, golf, biking, and skiing are all fair "game" for most people with diabetes. Heed a few words to the wise to get the most out of them and make them safer and more enjoyable.

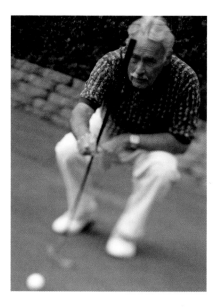

Take turns riding in the golf cart. Walking for the duration of your golf match will give you the most aerobic exercise, of course. But some walking is better than none. If you need to ride a cart at least part of the way, strike a deal with your partner to alternate who gets to drive, and who gets to walk. For instance, you might ride in the cart while playing one hole, and your partner would ride during the next hole.

If you're playing all 18 holes, prepare yourself for blood sugar swings. Before you start a round of golf—or any other sport that will keep you moving for the better part of the afternoon—be ready with a glucose meter, carbohydrate snacks or glucose tablets, and any medicine you might need to keep your blood sugar in the safe range.

After squash, check for *rising* glucose. Don't assume that all types of exercise will lower your blood sugar. In some people with diabetes, high-adrenaline sports, or any very strenuous exercise, can actually raise it. That's because adrenaline causes the liver to release more glucose to supply the body with a burst of energy. The effect does wear off, of course, and you should be ready for a possible drop in blood sugar up to several hours after you're done exercising. Regular testing—before, during, and after exercise—will help you determine how to manage your blood sugar levels with food, glucose, or insulin.

Before a tennis match, inject insulin into your abdomen, not your tennis arm. During heavy exercise, blood flow increases in the appendages that are working hard. If you inject insulin into a hard-working appendage, the insulin will be absorbed into the body more quickly, and it may lower your blood sugar more quickly than you were expecting. Same goes for runners—don't inject insulin into a leg before you hit the bricks.

Play on clay, not asphalt or concrete. Tennis can be tough on your hips, knees, ankles, and back. The repeated impact against a hard-court surface can leave your joints sore and your feet battered. Asphalt and concrete

Choosing the Safest Sport for *You*

If you have diabetes, exercise is your friend for a whole host of reasons. But you may need to choose one sport over another if you have certain other health problems related to diabetes. Here are a few general guidelines. Talk to your doctor about your own personal health situation and the activities you want to do.

If You Have Heart Disease

✔ Good for you
Moderate, non-strenuous activity in moderate temperatures. Try mall walking, swimming, or cycling on a stationary bike.

✖ Possibly unsafe
Straining and strenuous activity in very hot and humid weather or very cold weather. Avoid push-ups, sit-ups, and walking up steep hills.

If You Have Peripheral Arterial Disease

✔ Good for you
Aquatic exercise, cycling, and walking.

✖ Possibly unsafe
Weight-bearing and high-impact exercise such as basketball and tennis.

If You Have High Blood Pressure

✔ Good for you
Moderate aerobic and strength training exercise. Walking, jogging, and stair climbing are fine.

✖ Possibly unsafe
Straining and strenuous exercise, such as power-lifting with weights.

If You Have Neuropathy

✔ Good for you
Moderate intensity, low-impact exercises in moderate temperatures. Swimming is a good choice if you have pain or burning in your feet.

✖ Possibly unsafe
Strenuous, weight-bearing exercises such as step aerobics or hiking long distances and working out in extreme temperatures.

If You Have Retinopathy

✔ Good for you
Moderate, low-impact exercise with no straining during which you keep your head above your waist.

✖ Possibly unsafe
Anything that involves straining, jumping, holding your breath during exertion, or exercising with your head below waist level. Examples: Basketball, heavy weight lifting, and certain yoga poses.

If You Have Kidney Disease

✔ Good for you
Light or moderate exercise (such as walking or swimming) and high-repetition strength training (using light weights and doing more than 15 repetitions at a time).

✖ Possibly unsafe
High-intensity, vigorous sports and lifting heavy weights.

courts are the worst offenders. Studies show that clay courts have the lowest injury rates—they're softer, allow a little sliding underfoot so there's less shock to the feet, and they slow the game down to a less hectic level. New synthetic court surfaces provide cushioning that protects your joints, too—you can feel the surface give underneath your feet when you walk on it. Natural grass courts (like those at Wimbledon) are softer but have a high rate of injury because the speed of play is faster on grass.

Make sure that your diabetes gear is secure when bicycling long distances. Zippered pockets, a zipped-up backpack, and saddlebags with snug closures are good bets. You don't want to find yourself five miles from home on your bicycle and in need of a snack to keep your blood sugar up only to find that your food slipped out of your pocket.

Don't dally on hot surfaces. If you have reduced feeling in your feet, take care not to stand too long on sun-heated surfaces such as hard-surface

Can Exercise Reduce Your Need for Medication?

Regular physical activity doesn't just help you lose weight, burn fat, and feel great—it can actually lower your cells' resistance to insulin, a core problem in type 2 diabetes. The better your cells respond to insulin, the less medication you may need to take. If you're being diligent about following a new fitness plan and your blood sugar readings are showing a difference, it's worth talking to your doctor about whether you can reduce the number or quantity of medications you take.

Before your doctor agrees to make changes to your medications, she'll likely want to study your blood sugar log and see how different combinations of food, medication, and physical activity affect your blood sugar. The more details you can give your doctor about how you feel at any given time of the day, and what you did or ate before you took your reading, the better—a high blood sugar reading after exercise and a high reading after eating a jelly doughnut mean very different things.

If you use insulin, ask your doctor whether and when you can substitute exercise for an injection, or at least reduce the amount of insulin that you take before a workout. Ask her how to coordinate your physical activity with your food intake based on your blood sugar and insulin levels. Otherwise, you may run the risk of dangerously low blood glucose (hypoglycemia) or dangerously high blood glucose (hyperglycemia). Routinely checking your blood sugar before, during, and after physical activity will help you gauge, for example, when you'll need a snack break or how long to wait to exercise after taking insulin.

tennis courts, concrete pool areas, asphalt, and sand. Even through footwear, your feet could get burned without you knowing it.

Carry insulin and other gear under your ski jacket. To prevent your test strips and the insulin in your pump or vials from freezing while you are skiing, stash them close to your skin under your ski pants or jacket. One simple way to do this: Wear shorts that have a secure pocket under your ski pants, and slide your insulin and test strips into the pocket to keep them out of the deep freeze.

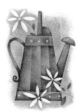

Always protect your eyes with sunglasses when exercising outdoors.

Buy custom-fitted ski boots. If you love skiing and you have reduced feeling in your feet, buy your own ski boots and take care that you get them fitted properly. When you rent ski boots, your odds of getting an excellent fit are awfully low. And if you're wearing ill-fitted boots and you have reduced sensation in your feet, you might not realize that your feet are being rubbed raw. If you have impaired circulation in your feet, ask your doctor whether skiing could cut off circulation to your feet or put you at risk for frostbite.

Wear sunglasses with UVA/UVB protection. Good sunglasses will protect your eyes from glare as well as the damaging rays in sunlight, which can contribute to cataracts—and people with diabetes are already 60 percent more likely to develop cataracts than people who do not have diabetes.

Carry a doctor's note clearing you for "extreme" sports. If you love some of the wilder sports such as white-water rafting, bungee jumping, or skydiving, take along a letter from your doctor stating that you are cleared for the activity. The operators of such sporting facilities often will ask whether you have diabetes and may refuse to admit you unless you can provide a doctor's approval. Without such a letter, you may end up cooling your heels for a few hours while your friends have the time of their lives.

Join a team. Whether it's tennis, volleyball, basketball, badminton, or paintball that floats your boat, get on the Internet and find a local team or league to join. Team sports not only boost fitness but self-esteem, too. And they're harder to quit than activities you do by yourself.

in the water

If you're overweight, or if you have joint or balance problems, foot pain from nerve damage, or other physical limitations—all of which are common among people who have diabetes—the swimming pool is a great place to get active. Since your weight is "reduced" by 90 percent in the water, swimming gives overweight people the buoyancy they need to keep their aerobic sessions going longer and move their bodies in ways they might not be able to do otherwise. Swimming is excellent aerobic exercise with an added benefit over walking: It exercises both the upper and lower body.

Splash in class. A water aerobics class may be the best way to get a full-body workout in the pool—and you don't even need to know how to swim. If there's upbeat music playing and you're with a nice group of people, you may even feel a little bit like you're at a party. Want to get competitive? Your pool might have a recreational water volleyball team, so call and inquire.

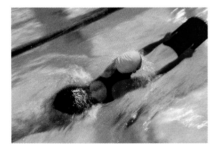

Get a leg up with a kickboard. Your buoyancy in the water is already protecting your joints from impact, but if you need even more lift, a kickboard will help. They're also handy if you're not confident of your swimming ability and want extra help in staying afloat. People who just want to exercise their legs can grab a kickboard by its sides and propel themselves through the water with leg power.

Work up to a 30-minute swim. Swim one pool length (25 meters in a standard pool), and then rest for 30 seconds. If that didn't challenge you, alternate swimming for 5 minutes and resting for 1 minute. Each time you visit the pool, add gradually to your swimming distance, resting as needed, until you reach 30 minutes of total swim time each session. To steadily improve your aerobic fitness, swim three times a week.

If your sight is impaired, ask about "lap time." Many pools set aside times exclusively for lane swimming, during which swim lanes are roped off and recreational swimmers splashing around are prohibited. Having your own designated lane reduces the chances that you'll collide with someone you couldn't see coming.

Protect wounds while in the water. Swimming when you have an open wound isn't a good idea because it increases your risk of infection. Rather than skipping your aqua-workout when you have a cut or sore, ask your doctor whether a waterproof bandage or another skin barrier is appropriate for your situation. Be sure to clear the bandage with the pool's lifeguard or manager before you jump in.

Be extra-alert for low blood sugar symptoms. It may harder when you're in a pool to tell if you're sweating or feeling weak so be vigilant, and get out of the pool if you can as soon as you suspect a problem.

Get clearance to keep food near the pool. If your blood sugar drops while you're in the water, you may not have time to get out and go to your locker to reach your snack. So keep a high-carbohydrate snack in a zip-close plastic bag poolside while you swim. If the pool has rules against keeping food near the water, talk to the lifeguard, pool manager, or your water aerobics instructor and explain your needs—they will probably make an exception, or at least will allow you to keep glucose tablets or gel handy.

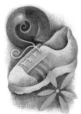

Keep your insulin pump cool on shore. If you're at the beach or an outdoor pool on a warm day and you want to disconnect your insulin pump and swim, keep the pump cool so the insulin doesn't deteriorate. Place the insulin pump in a zip-close plastic bag, wrap a small towel around it, and place it in a cooler. Alternatively, check with your pump's manufacturer to see if it offers a special protective, waterproof pouch for your model.

Wearing water shoes or aqua socks when you swim will help prevent injuries.

If you swim with your pump, recognize its limits. Some insulin pumps are advertised as being "waterproof" (sometimes with the use of inserts to plug the vent holes), but read the instructions carefully about the limits of this protection. The waterproofing may only apply to near-the-surface use and may not apply if you're diving more than about nine feet underwater. If you find that the tape on your infusion set keeps coming loose in the water, pick up a very lightweight wet suit T-shirt and wear that over the infusion set. The close-fitting shirt will prevent water from peeling up the edges of the tape.

Shower immediately after swimming. Otherwise, the chlorine from the pool water will dry out your skin and might cause it to crack, which will make you more vulnerable to infection.

Protect your feet in lakes and oceans—even in pools. People with diabetes are prone to slower healing, and serious infections in the feet can even lead to amputation. Wearing water shoes or aqua socks when you're swimming in a lake or ocean will help prevent injuries from rocks, sea life, glass, or other debris. Wearing protection in man-made swimming areas isn't a bad idea either; the concrete floors of some pools are abrasive.

Apply water-resistant sunscreen when you swim outside. The water may feel cool against your skin, but you could still get burned under the hot sun, even on overcast days. Sunburn is not healthy for anyone, but it's particularly vexing for people with diabetes because it can take longer to heal and, if it's bad, could possibly raise your blood sugar.

pool exercise

There are plenty of effective ways to get an aerobic workout in the swimming pool without swimming a stroke—and your joints will be spared the pounding that they would suffer on land. Position yourself in a part of the pool where the water level is between your hips and your armpits. As you take steps during these exercises, place your whole foot flat against the bottom of the pool. Wear water shoes for better traction and to protect your feet.

1 | walking or running

The same movements that get your heart pumping on land will give you a workout in the water, too—with less danger of stumbling. **Bend** your arms at the elbow and **pump** them forward and back as you go. **Alternate** walking (or running) forward, then backward.

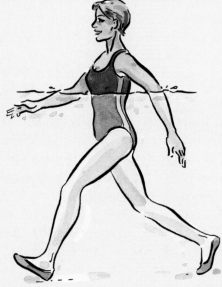

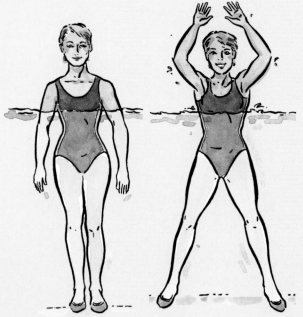

2 | jumping jacks

It's just as you learned in grade school: **Start** by standing in the pool with your legs together and your hands at your sides. **Jump** and **spread** your feet to shoulder width while you raise your hands up to touch over your head. Jump again and return to the starting position.

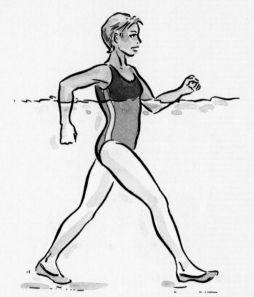

3 | cross-country skiing

This exercise is done standing in place. Start by standing in the pool, with your right leg forward and your left leg behind you. **Hop** slightly and **reverse** leg positions—left leg forward and right leg back. **Pump** your arms at your sides as you move your legs.

4 | front kick

Wrap a flexible foam water noodle around your back for extra support. **Begin** by standing in the pool. **Raise** your left leg in front of you, then return to the standing position. Repeat with the right.

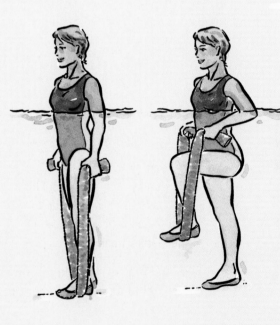

5 | knee lift

Stand up straight with the noodle under your left foot. Bending the leg, **lift** your left knee to hip level, moving the noodle as you go. Return to starting position. Repeat with the right.

on your feet

Whether it's strolling on the beach that stirs your soul or walking every square foot of a flea market, moving your feet is doing your body good, so keep it up. If you're doing something you love, you won't even notice how much ground you're covering.

Hit flea markets and antique shops. Grab your calendar and schedule one day of leisurely browsing. Daydream about where you'd like to go, and make it happen: Maybe it's ambling through a cluster of antique shops that you've been meaning to visit, picking through the tables at a flea market, or strolling up and down your favorite row of quaint shops. If you're on a tight budget, no problem—leave your money at home.

Get lost in a large garden or gorgeous park. Maybe you can't resist inspecting every wild plant you see or snapping photos of the nature around you. Either way, terrific! Bringing your hobby with you as you walk turns "riding the shoe leather" into a satisfying, stress-relieving outing. Don't forget to bring your bird log if you're a birder.

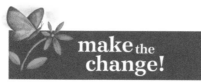

The habit: Bumping up walks to 90 minutes a day.

The result: Reduction of A1C blood sugar scores by 1.1 percent—and possibly reducing the insulin or other medications you take.

The proof: In a two-year study of people with type 2 diabetes, those who walked for 90 minutes a day reduced their A1C scores (a measure of long-term blood sugar control) by an average of 1.1 percent. The number of these people who needed to take insulin dropped by 25 percent, and those who remained on insulin reduced their usage by an average of 11 units per day. Yes, 90 minutes is a lot of exercise, but shorter walks were also beneficial: Study subjects who walked for 38 minutes per day still reduced their A1C scores by an average of 0.4 percent.

Take a dog or a child along. If you're giving a dog a chance to lap up the outdoors or a child a new view on the nature show before her, you're doing much more than mere walking. The time will pass more quickly, you'll walk longer—and you'll come back with spirits lifted.

Mind your posture. Carrying yourself correctly can alleviate joint pain (and make you look thinner and taller). Stand erect with your shoulders up, your stomach muscles tightened, and your chin up. Tilt forward slightly from the waist. Bend your arms at the elbow and pump them as you walk. End each step you take by pushing off with your toes.

Calculate how fast you're walking and set a goal to speed up. Drive along your favorite walking route until you have measured out one mile on your car's odometer. The next time you walk, time yourself as you walk that mile. (You might walk more than that one mile, but this is the spot to check your pace.) If it took you 20 minutes, pick up the pace a little the next day and see if you can complete the mile in 19 minutes. As a point of reference: A 15- to 20-minute mile is considered a brisk walk.

chapter eight

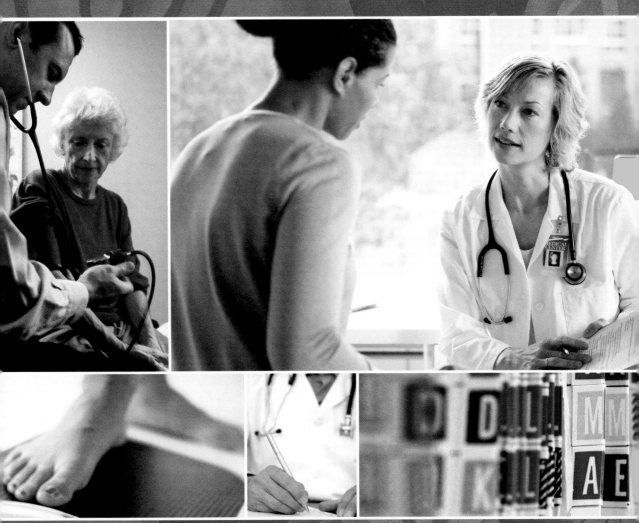

at the doctor's office

You're the one ultimately in charge of your diabetes day to day, but your doctor is your trusty guide, whom you'll turn to for medications, tests, and expert advice. The better your partnership is, the better your diabetes management will be.

working with your doctor

While you probably won't be having dinner dates with your doctor, he or she can be your best friend when it comes to helping you manage your diabetes. So open your arms and be ready to embrace (figuratively speaking) that relationship, and help your doctor help you.

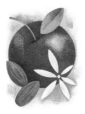

Be prepared to talk about what you've been eating and how much you're exercising.

Befriend the support staff. It never hurts to say a friendly word to the people who work with your physician. Office administrators, physician's assistants, and nurses can be extremely helpful when it comes to getting more face time with your doctor, answering questions about insurance coverage, or providing you a quick answer when your doctor isn't available. It's also a good idea to be considerate by arriving on time and giving at least 24 hours notice if you need to reschedule an appointment.

Keep up with your doctor visits. Waiting too long between doctor visits and assuming everything will stay the same in the interim is like driving blindfolded and assuming that the road is straight. Most people with diabetes visit the doctor every three to four months, but that can vary depending on your health status, including your glucose levels and how stable they are. Ask your doctor how often she'd like to see you, and keep those appointments. If you go for long periods without seeing your doctor and your glucose is not under control, you could cause yourself some serious trouble.

Bring your glucose log book and your food log if you keep one. The best way your doctor can help you mange your blood sugar is to sit down with you and take a look at both of these tools, help you pin down the food factors that seem to be influencing your blood sugar, and point out ways to change them for the better. Unfortunately, not all general practitioners will take the time—or even have the expertise—to do this. If you're not getting enough help along these lines, you'll want to see a registered dietitian or a certified diabetes educator (see page 150). Also be prepared to talk about what kind of exercise you've been doing. If you haven't been doing a lick, seeing that doctor's appointment on the calendar may spur you to lace up those sneakers.

Bring an extra set of ears. The average doctor's appointment lasts less than seven minutes. Sometimes it's hard to take everything in. If possible, bring someone with you to just listen to what the doctor says. After the appointment, compare notes. Also, if you wear hearing aids, don't forget to wear them. If you don't have anyone to bring with you, you may be able to find an advocate from a diabetes support group (look for groups at your local hospital or search www.diabetes.org) to accompany you.

Wear comfortable clothing and shoes that can be easily removed. It seems like a simple suggestion, but having lots of buttons or laces can make getting undressed for examinations cumbersome. Loose pants with an elastic waist, a comfy T-shirt or sweater, and slip-on shoes are perfect.

Take off your socks and shoes even if your doctor doesn't tell you to. Your feet should be examined at every visit for signs of skin breakdown, hot spots, cracked heals, or ingrown toenails.

Put your log book between your toes. This way you'll be sure that both your feet and your log book will be examined!

Ask what your blood pressure is. Sometimes doctors take your blood pressure and don't tell you the result—but you should know. Ideally, blood pressure for people with diabetes should be 130/80 or lower. If your pressure is higher, it means your heart is working too hard and can indicate an increased risk of heart disease, stroke, and nerve and kidney damage.

Take a few deep breaths before he checks your blood pressure. This will help you get a more accurate reading, especially if you tend to get a little nervous in the doctor's office. Make sure your feet are flat on the floor.

Bring a list of all medications and supplements you take. Don't forget to list over-the-counter medications, vitamins, and herbs, in addition to prescription drugs. This will help your doctor quickly determine if you're taking two things that interact badly, or if you're taking something you really don't need. It will also clue him in to side effects that may be related to something you're taking.

Know Your Blood Sugar Goals

Ideally, you'll strive to get your blood sugar as close to the normal (nondiabetic) range as possible. These are the general guidelines from the American Diabetes Association.

• **Normal blood sugar:** Generally speaking, glucose levels should be between 90 and 130 mg/dl before meals, and less than 180 mg/dl two hours after starting a meal. Your doctor will work with you to come up with specific targets, either higher or lower, for you.

• **High blood sugar:** Too high is anything over 140 mg/dl before a meal, or higher than 160 mg/dl at bedtime.

• **When to call your doctor:** Ask your doctor what is too high for you. Typically you'll need to call your doctor anytime your blood sugar is over 250 mg/dl.

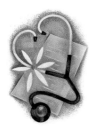

Make sure your doctor's recommendations and goals are realistic for your life.

Learn how to get help after office hours. Is there an alternate number you should call? Who are the other doctors who will be on call when your doctor is out of town? Which emergency room should you use? Ask these questions *before* a crisis strikes.

Need a new doctor? Gather word-of-mouth recommendations. Ask for referrals from friends, people you know who have diabetes, or your doctor. Do a bit of digging about why a friend is suggesting a doctor. Does she listen well? Is he experienced in working with people with diabetes? Can you get in to see her quickly?

Have a get-to-know-you visit. If you've located a doctor who looks promising, see if you can make an initial appointment before committing (some insurance carriers won't cover this, but it's worth checking). You can get a feel for how you mesh with the physician and how busy and how organized the office is.

Make sure your diabetes plan is a good fit for you. Speak up if for any reason you have concerns about your doctor's recommendations and expectations—for example, if your feet burn so much that you can't exercise, if you're having trouble getting rides to your doctor's appointments, if you are terrified of needles and don't think you can inject yourself with insulin, or there's nowhere to refrigerate your insulin at work. These are all problems your doctor can help you solve or work around.

When doctor shopping, ask leading questions. Does she have a large number of patients with diabetes? (More diabetes patients means more experience treating people with diabetes.) Does she refer diabetes patients for diabetes education? What target blood sugar numbers does she consider acceptable? Can she tell you what her average A1C (a long-term measure of blood sugar control) number is for her patients with diabetes? (Normal is 4 to 6 percent mg/dl; the goal for people with diabetes should be under 7 percent, or under 6 percent according to some sources.) Does she use electronic medical records? (Studies show that MDs who keep electronic records keep better track of the tests their patients need.) Answers to these questions will tell you a lot about her experience with diabetes care.

Does Your Doctor Have a Bald Spot?

If your doctor has a computer in the exam room and you find that he spends more time looking at it than you, you need to take action. You might think this is bold, but get up and look over his shoulder to see what is so interesting. You'll make your point.

before your appointment

You probably see your doctor only a handful of times each year, so make the most of those visits with a little advance preparation. It could pay off later by eliminating the hassle of having to repeat an appointment because of a missed lab test or because you forgot to ask an important question.

Make a list of questions. Doctor visits go by so fast that it's hard to remember everything you wanted to ask or mention unless you write it down. To make sure you keep track of each question, number or bullet each item on your list, leave space to take notes, and check off each item after you've talked it over. That way, even if you get sidetracked, you'll be able to refer back to your notes to know what still needs to be discussed.

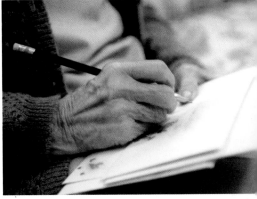

Get lab tests done in plenty of time before your visit. Your doctor may ask you to have tests prior to your appointment, and if you wait till the last minute, you may not get your results in time for your appointment.

Get detailed instructions for upcoming lab work. Find out if you'll need to make an appointment at the lab, or if they have walk-in times. Will you need to refrain from eating or drinking prior to the test or wear comfortable shoes and clothes if you're going for an exercise stress test? Do you need to have lab work completed a certain number of days before your appointment?

Review your diet. Truth be told, if you're not careful, you can "out-eat" the effectiveness of most diabetes drugs. Before your next visit, take an honest look at your diet and ask yourself if you're doing everything you can to eat better foods on a better schedule. At what times of day do you generally eat? (Many diabetes medications are more effective when properly timed with meals.) How often do you eat out? (It's much harder to keep calories under control when you eat outside your house.) What are your portion sizes—small, medium, large, or immense? Do you limit sugary or high-fat foods? Your doctor will probably ask about your food habits; if not, ask him if he would like to know what you eat and when you eat it.

Maintain your normal eating and drinking routine. That is, unless your doctor told you to fast. (If you're not sure, call your doctor's office at least 24 hours before your next appointment and ask.) If you're eating or drinking habits were out of the ordinary in any way on the day of an appointment or lab test, be sure to tell your doctor because that could cause an altered heart rate, blood pressure, or test results.

questions to ask

Simply being in a doctor's office can be intimidating. And most doctors don't have much time to spend with patients, so it's not uncommon to feel a bit rushed. But don't stifle your questions. Getting the answers you need makes the difference between taking good care of your diabetes, and your health in general, and letting it slip from your control. Start with the tips here.

How often should I check my blood sugar? The answer will depend on several factors. See "How Often Should You Check Your Blood Sugar?" on page 148. At each visit, you'll want to review and discuss how you are using your monitoring results at home and whether you should increase or decrease your monitoring schedule.

How and when do I take my medications? This is critical, and the instructions for you might be different than for somebody else, so pay careful attention, and take notes. Make sure you know if you should take your medication or insulin before or after meals, at night or in the morning, with or without food, etcetera. Do you need to avoid alcohol? Are there potential interactions with other drugs that you should know about? This information will be in the bag when you pick up your prescription, but the language can be hard to understand, so it doesn't hurt to ask while you're in the office.

Is there a generic version of my medication? If money is a concern, ask about drug alternatives. Sometimes a doctor can switch you to an older drug that's equally effective and less costly or to a generic version of the drug.

What side effects could I experience? Any prescription you receive should come with a patient pamphlet that describes possible side effects and symptoms, but it's smart to discuss these issues when the doctor first prescribes your medications. Are some side effects more likely than others? Will the medication make you drowsy or unable to drive a car? What symptoms warrant a call to the doctor? Should you stop taking a drug if

golden rule! ## See Your Doctor as an Equal

All those certificates and diplomas on the doctor's wall can be very impressive and intimidating ... but does he know how to change a spark plug, fix a gourmet meal, speak a second language, or paint? Remind yourself that you have talents that he doesn't have, and that he has talents that you may not have. One person is not better than the other. Keep this in mind and you may not be as intimidated or shy about asking questions.

you experience certain unpleasant effects? If for any reason you do stop taking a medication, call you doctor and let him know right away. Don't wait for the next appointment.

What sort of eating plan should I follow? For a real answer to this question, you'll want a referral to a registered dietitian (see page 150), since most MDs are not very well trained in nutrition. In the meantime, it's still a good idea to ask your doctor for general guidelines. Most doctors' offices have pamphlets that give healthy eating suggestions for people with diabetes. Typically this will involve not skipping meals, eating at the same times of day every day, eating about the same amounts of food at a given mealtime, and focusing on fresh fruits and vegetables, whole grains, low-fat dairy, and lean protein foods.

Can I drink alcohol? If you choose to drink alcohol, the general guideline is no more than one drink a day for an adult woman and a maximum of two drinks per day for an adult man. (One drink is 5 ounces of wine or one 12-ounce beer.) If your doctor has concerns about your kidneys or liver, he may suggest that you abstain from alcohol.

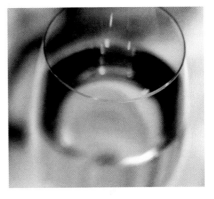

Should I avoid certain foods? Based on your blood pressure, cholesterol, and blood sugar averages, your doctor may suggest some dietary changes. The prevailing school of thought is that you can still enjoy most of the foods you enjoyed before being diagnosed with diabetes, including sweets, though maybe not in the same amounts or prepared in the same way. Some habits, though, like drinking several cans of regular soda per day (which have the equivalent of 12 teaspoons of sugar each), will probably have to change.

Am I clear for bungee jumping or basketball? As long as you don't have serious health complications, most doctors will recommend moderate exercise such as walking, swimming, or riding a bike for 30 minutes most days a week. Still, it is a good idea to get the go-ahead from your physician if you're starting a new physical activity or exercise regimen. He may want to give you a physical or at least consider your condition (whether you have kidney disease, nerve damage, signs of heart disease, or other problems) before giving you the A-okay.

Can I reduce any of my medications? This is a good question to ask if you've been eating well and exercising religiously, and you've seen significant improvements in your blood sugar numbers as a result.

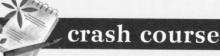

diabetes medications

A healthy diet and exercise will always be critical to keeping your diabetes under control—but it won't always be enough. There will likely come a time, if it hasn't come already, that your doctor will prescribe pills or insulin to help you control your blood sugar. Here's a primer on what you can expect.

who needs drugs?

At first, your doctor may try to have you bring down your blood sugar by improving your diet and adding regular exercise, but the percentage of people who can stay off medications by eating better and exercising is low.

If your blood sugar is dangerously high, your doctor may start you off on medications, then work with you to lower your blood sugar levels with lifestyle measures—he can reduce or stop your medications later if your levels improve. You may also be prescribed drugs early on if you are someone who isn't overweight (about 10 percent of people with type 2 diabetes are a healthy weight), or if you already are eating well and exercising regularly. Even if you don't fall into one of these categories, it's becoming more common for doctors to prescribe an oral drug such as metformin right from the start. (According to estimates, most people have had diabetes for at least five years before they are diagnosed, so this makes sense.)

Even if you don't start off using medications, many people will eventually need drug therapy. The longer you have diabetes, the harder it is to manage it with diet and exercise alone.

what about insulin?

Sometimes it makes sense to use insulin right away. This can be especially true if you have extremely high blood sugar levels at the time of diagnosis or if you have severe liver or kidney

damage, or a greater need for insulin due to illness or stress. Still, most people start with one or two oral medications. If it becomes obvious that diet, exercise, and pills aren't working, your doctor may decide that it is time for insulin.

how does my doctor decide what medications I need?

There are a handful of different kinds of diabetes drugs available, and your doctor may use them alone or in combination, depending on what sort of help your body needs to control your blood sugar. Some drugs work on the pancreas to help your body secrete more insulin; some lower the amount of stored sugar released from your liver; some lower your cells' resistance to insulin; some help your body release a quick burst of insulin when you eat; and some slow down the rate at which carbohydrates reach your bloodstream after a meal. Certain drugs, called sulfonylureas, can cause weight gain, so your doctor may avoid prescribing one of these if you're overweight. Your doctor will also consider your kidney function; drugs that are eliminated from the body through the kidneys, such as metformin, may not be a good choice for you if you have kidney damage.

can I use inhaled insulin?

The first powdered inhalable insulin, Exubera, was introduced in 2006. It freed some people with diabetes from having to use needles at all and helped others to reduce the number of pills and injections they required. In 2007, Pfizer stopped making the drug due to economic (not safety) reasons, but it's likely that another drug company will step in and fill the void. You may be able to use inhaled insulin in place of some diabetes pills, mealtime insulin, or in combination with oral medications or longer-acting insulin. Besides hypoglycemia, other potential side effects include dry mouth, coughing, chest discomfort, and decreased lung capacity. Before your doctor prescribes inhaled insulin, she should test your lung capacity with a spirometry test. If you smoke, have lung disease or asthma, or have quit smoking less than six months ago, you shouldn't use inhaled insulin.

why does my doctor change my dose or my drug?

Because diabetes is a progressive disease, over time, most drugs, including insulin, become less effective the longer you take them. Your doctor may increase your levels of medication if he sees them becoming less effective. Or he may change your regimen altogether if you aren't seeing good results from your current one.

what are the side effects and risks of drugs?

In general, diabetes medications are safe and work well. But like any other drugs, they have potential side effects. Discuss specifics of each of your medications with your doctor, and read the package insert when you pick up your prescription. Any drug can interact with other medicines—prescription or otherwise—and some diabetes pills do not sit well with alcohol, so be sure to get good directions and heed them. Common side effects of some drugs are hypoglycemia, stomach upset, skin reactions, bloating, and weight gain. Certain drugs, over time, can damage your liver. And in 2007, the FDA added a "black box warning," its toughest warning, on prescription labels for rosiglitazone (Avandia) because it may increase the risk of congestive heart failure. Check for a black box warning on any drug you've been prescribed, and if there is one, have a discussion with your doctor about it.

Drug Treatments for Type 2 Diabetes

Your doctor's approach may vary. All treatments include diet and exercise.

BLOOD SUGAR NUMBERS	LIKELY TREATMENT APPROACH	EXPECTED A1C DROP	COMMENTS
A1C <8% Fasting glucose <200 mg/dl	Weight loss if overweight, exercise, dietary changes, and possibly an oral drug	1% after 3 months (for diet and exercise alone)	Trend is toward prescribing an oral drug right at diagnosis.
A1C 8–8.9% Fasting glucose 200–250 mg/dl	One or more oral or injectable (non-insulin) drugs	1–2% after 1–3 months	Oral drugs are ineffective past their maximum dose; adding another drug can help.
A1C 8–8.9% Fasting glucose 251–300 mg/dl	Three-drug therapy	2–4% after 1–3 months	This can be expensive and inconvenient. Insulin may be a better choice.
A1C 8–8.9% Fasting glucose >300 mg/dl	Insulin	Unlimited	Insulin is needed when beta cells stop producing insulin or cells are extremely insulin resistant.

share your symptoms

Some of us hold back on letting our doctors know the little details of how we've been feeling, hiding that swollen toe under a sock, or "forgetting" to mention new problems in the bedroom. But it's essential to speak up because what seems like a harmless bit of indigestion, an extra dry spot on your skin, a "floater" in your eye, or tingling in the feet could indicate something more serious than you think.

Be clear when explaining symptoms. Instead of just telling your doctor, "I've been feeling lousy," try to be as specific as possible. For example, "I've been feeling a tingling in my feet for the last two weeks." Describe your symptoms as precisely as possible, say what you've been doing to relieve them (if anything), and note whether anything seems to help reduce them. The more specific your description, the easier it will be for your doctor to figure out a diagnosis and treatment.

Report any tingling, numbness, burning, or pain. These sensations in your feet, legs, arms, or hands can be a sign of nerve damage, or neuropathy. The feelings often start in the feet and can be slight at first. Tell your doctor if you have any sensitivity to touch, leg cramps, difficulty sensing the position of you feet, or feelings of being off-balance. Other markers of circulation and nerve problems in the feet are sores, blisters, or cracks that won't heal.

Scale your pain. It might be helpful to tell your doctor how much pain or discomfort you are in by using a scale of 1 to 10, where 10 is excruciating pain and 1 is very mild discomfort.

Share even embarrassing symptoms. While you may feel uncomfortable talking about frequent urination or erectile dysfunction, doctors hear about these problems all the time.

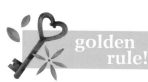

golden rule! Know the Signs of High and Low Blood Sugar

Common signs and symptoms of hypo-glycemia (low blood sugar) are confusion, hunger, weakness, shakiness, perspiration, rapid heart beat, dizziness, nervousness, or irritability. Signs and symptoms of hyper-glycemia (high blood sugar) include, fatigue, thirst, frequent urination, blurry vision, hunger, and sudden weight loss. You won't necessarily have all the symptoms at the same time, and symptoms can vary from episode to episode. Some people report unusual symptoms such as their nose going numb or their ears ringing. If you find this to be true for you, let your doctor in on your discovery.

learn to monitor your blood sugar effectively

The whole point of taking medications, eating healthy foods in moderate portions, and exercising is to keep your blood sugar within reasonable targets—and there's no way to know how well these steps are working without checking your blood sugar regularly. The more often you test, the better you can hone in on the perfect combination of strategies.

Master the self-test. Your doctor or someone in his office should demonstrate how to do a self-test. You'll start by sticking your finger with a small needle, called a lancet. Some meters have a built in lancet that takes blood from your forearm or thigh, and there are also spring-loaded lancing devices, that resemble a pen, that make sticking yourself less painful. If you use your fingertip, stick the side of your fingertip by your fingernail to avoid having sore spots on your finger pads. Apply the drop of blood to a testing strip. Your meter will provide results in about 5 to 30 seconds, and you'll record the numbers in a log book; some meters record and store the results.

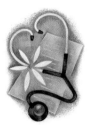

Ask your doctor what blood sugar level is too high and warrants a phone call.

Get specific directions on what times of day you should check blood sugar. Everyone's schedule will be different. See "How Often Should You Check Your Blood Sugar?" on the next page.

Discuss meter options with your doctor, and call your insurance company before making a purchase. Many cover some or all of the cost of meters and other supplies. You can also ask for a referral to a diabetes educator, who might have samples of meters available for you to see and touch.

Know what to do if your results are too low. If you get a result of 70 mg/dl or under, your blood sugar is too low and you should consume 15 grams of carbohydrate. Even if you feel okay, don't wait for the symptoms of hypoglycemia to kick in. Take three to four glucose tablets, ½ cup of orange juice, 1 tablespoon of honey, six Lifesaver candies, ¾ cup regular soda, or 1 tablespoon of sugar dissolved in water. (A candy bar isn't ideal because the fat it contains can delay the glucose-raising effect.) Wait about 15 minutes, then check your blood sugar again.

Be prepared to bring down high blood sugar. First, clarify with your doctor what level is too high for you. It could be 250 mg/dl, or it could be higher. Whatever the cut-off point, you'll need to call your doctor if you hit it. You'll also need to alert your doctor's office if you have elevated readings (higher than your designated goals) for more than three days in a row. Often, illness, stress, missing a dose of medication, or eating too much can cause spikes in your blood sugar.

Address high morning blood sugar. During the wee hours of the morning, the body secretes hormones that inhibit insulin so that more glucose is available to the body at the start of the day—not what you need if you have diabetes. A related phenomenon can happen if your blood sugar drops too low in the middle of the night, causing your body to react—actually, to over-react—by releasing hormones that raise blood sugar. If you notice a pattern of high morning blood sugar, talk to your doctor. You may need to change the type or dosage of medication or insulin you take, or when you take it, or tweak your evening eating habits. Your blood glucose will be easier to manage throughout the day if you can start the day off with normal readings.

Know when to check more often. You'll want to do extra checks when you're sick or under significant stress. Your doctor may also request that you do extra checks when you make a change to your treatment plan.

How Often Should You Check Your Blood Sugar?

The point of checking your blood sugar is to see what effect the foods you are eating, the medications you are taking, and the exercise you are doing have on your levels, so you can tell how well they're working. The more often you check, the more information you'll have. Here are general guidelines.

If you aren't taking oral medications or insulin, your doctor will most likely recommend that you check your glucose levels in the morning and before dinner, and possibly at bedtime, either daily or occasionally. This will tell him what your blood sugar is when you start your day and how the meals you eat during the day affect you. If by nightfall your blood sugars are in the target range, that means your blood sugars most likely have stayed in target range. An A1C test will confirm if this is so.

If you are taking oral medications, your doctor will probably recommend checking more often—maybe before certain meals and two hours after the start of a meal. This regimen will tell him what your blood sugar is going into the meal and what effect your meal has on your blood sugar. He can use this information to adjust your medications or give you some dietary advice to get your blood sugar back in target range.

If you are taking insulin, your doctor will likely have you check before meals and occasionally after meals and at bedtime. (If you are taking Lantus, a once-a-day "background" insulin, you may not be asked to check before each meal. This insulin is adjusted according to morning fasting blood sugar levels.) If you wake up in the morning sweaty, with the bed sheets all askew, and you've have had a bad dream, you may have experienced low blood sugar in the middle of the night. Your doctor may ask you to set your alarm and check your blood sugar at 3 a.m. to see if you are experiencing hypoglycemia in the middle of the night.

build a strong health care team

Your regular doctor may be the one watching over your diabetes in general, but your feet, kidneys, eyes—even your diet and exercise—will need extra-special TLC because diabetes affects your whole body. In fact, it takes a team of people to properly manage diabetes, so work with your doctor to put one in place.

For stubborn blood sugar, see a specialist. If your blood sugar readings aren't showing any improvement, even after following your doctor's advice closely for at least 12 to 16 weeks, ask to see a diabetes specialist, also referred to as a diabetologist. This is a doctor who specializes in treating people with diabetes and is usually also an endocrinologist. Not all endocrinologists specialize in diabetes, though, so it is important to ask before making an appointment.

Request a referral to a certified diabetes educator. This professional, usually a registered nurse, dietitian, or pharmacist, has specialized diabetes training and will have more time to spend with you than your doctor. He or she can help you adopt, adapt, and adhere to the better behaviors that will help improve your blood sugar control. This person can answer questions about your medications, show you how to give yourself insulin shots, help you check blood sugar effectively, suggest better ways to keep track of your blood sugar records, and more. Many are employed in a Diabetes Self-Management Education (DSME) program, and services from these programs are reimbursed by Medicare. If your doctor doesn't offer DSME in his office, ask for a referral for DSME, or call your local hospital to request diabetes education.

Make healthy eating habits a priority by seeing a registered dietitian (RD). What you eat and when you eat it affect your blood sugar more than any other lifestyle choice. If you have diabetes, you need an eating plan tailored just for you to help you meet your blood sugar goals. The person who can provide that plan is a registered dietician who specializes in helping people with diabetes. She'll help you figure out how much food you should be eating, learn portion control, understand healthy food choices, and plan meals that will fit your lifestyle. Not all registered dietitians specialize in diabetes, so make sure you are referred to one who does. Some RDs are also certified diabetes educators.

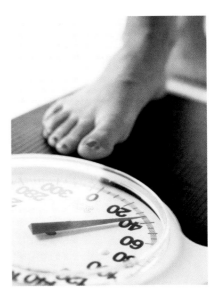

golden rule!　Keep—and Study—a Food Log

Itemizing each piece of food that passes your lips might seem like a pain, but it can do you some real good. It's easy to forget, or minimize, the snacking you did when you were making the lasagna for dinner, or the bite of blood-sugar-spiking birthday cake you couldn't resist at the office party. Unconscious habits and patterns become more obvious when you see them in print. Plus, knowing that you'll be reviewing a food diary with your registered dietitian or diabetes educator might give you the willpower to pass on the cake and pick up an apple instead.

If you saw a registered dietitian years ago, it's time to see one again. Even if you've had diabetes for many years, a visit with a nutritionist can be very helpful. Nutrition and calorie needs change with age, and guidelines for good nutrition may also have shifted since you were diagnosed. A visit with an RD can also renew your motivation to eat better. You may even go home with some fun new recipes to try.

See an ophthalmologist at least once a year. Chronic high blood sugar can damage blood vessels in your retina (the inner layer of the eyes), which increases your chances of vision disorders and even blindness, so you'll need to make sure you have an annual comprehensive eye exam with an ophthalmologist. He will dilate your eyes to enlarge your pupils and have an extra-close look for any changes in your eyes. If you are referred to a new eye doctor, be sure to ask if he is familiar with spotting and treating diabetic eye disorders.

See your dentist twice a year. You learned when you were a kid that sugar causes cavities. Well, having high blood sugar can wreak havoc on your teeth, too. Bacteria that cause gum disease and cavities are more opportunistic—that is, nastier—when blood sugar is not well controlled. That's why people with diabetes are more prone to gum disease, which, believe it or not, has been linked to an increased risk of heart disease. In addition to regular dental visits, you need to brush and floss daily. It also pays to check monthly for any sores, tenderness, or redness of your gums.

Bring your feet to an expert. It's awfully hard to imagine that a simple blister or cut could lead to foot amputation, but if the injury turns into an ulcer that becomes infected, it's all too possible. That's why it's critical to take good care of your feet. A podiatrist will check for any sores, blisters, bruises, cracks, or cuts that are resistant to healing, as well as check for tingling or numbness in your feet. He can confirm nerve problems by doing a variety of tests using a tuning fork against various body parts to see if you can detect vibrations, or by using heat or cold to see if you can detect these sensations. Discuss with your regular doctor how often you should see a podiatrist, and make sure to go to one who specializes in caring for people with diabetes. Your regular doctor should also check your feet at every visit.

When you visit your podiatrist, take the shoes you wear most often. The podiatrist can tell you whether your shoes are appropriate and whether you need any adjustments to your footwear, such as insoles or added padding. Do the doc a favor and air the shoes out the day before!

Four Common Diabetes Tests

Here's a cheat sheet on common tests your doctor may have you take.

A1C: This is a simple blood test done in a lab that shows your average blood sugar levels over the last three months. The test is usually performed every three to six months to give your doctor an idea of how well your diabetes treatment program is working. The blood can be drawn any time, regardless of what you've eaten. For people who do not have diabetes, a normal A1C is between 4 and 6 percent. Typically, you want to see a number that is less than 7 and as close to normal as possible. If your levels are too high, your doctor may alter your treatment plan to bring your blood sugar levels down. See the conversion chart on page 272 to learn how A1C numbers translate to the numbers you write in your blood sugar log.

Microalbuminuria: This is a urine test, usually performed annually, that shows how well your kidneys are functioning by measuring albumin, a protein whose presence indicates early stage kidney damage.

Creatinine: If there are concerns about kidney damage, your doctor may suggest this blood test. Creatinine is a waste product that is normally removed from the body by the kidneys, but as kidney disease progresses, the level of creatinine in the blood increases.

Cholesterol and triglycerides: This blood test, usually done annually, checks your levels of three kinds of fats. LDL, or "bad" cholesterol, is a waxy fat that can build up and harden on the walls of your arteries. Levels should be 100 mg/dl or less. HDL, or "good" cholesterol, is a healthy fat that actually removes the LDL from your veins and arteries. For people with diabetes, HDL should be above 50 mg/dl for women and 40 mg/dl for men. Triglycerides are the circulating storage form of fat, which your body produces from excess glucose or fat. Too much can cause hardening of the arteries. Your levels should be less than 150 mg/dl.

golden rule! Get a Yearly Flu Shot

People with diabetes are about three times as likely to die from the flu or pneumonia as people who don't have the disease, but only one-third of them ever get the available vaccinations. The American Diabetes Association recommends both shots for anyone ages two or older who has diabetes. One pneumonia vaccination is usually enough to protect for a lifetime, but some doctors will recommend that people with diabetes have a follow-up shot 5 to 10 years after their first one.

Request a referral to a personal trainer. More and more doctors are starting to work with, or recommend, personal trainers, exercise professionals who will work with you one-on-one to design a fitness program for you and help you meet your goals. But you need to express a willingness to go. If you really want to stick with an exercise program, a trainer can help tremendously if they have experience working with people with diabetes. (You should ask.) You can also check at your local hospital or diabetes support group for a recommendation.

Know when to ask for a counselor. Mental health professionals such as psychologists, social workers, or family counselors can offer additional support for dealing with the personal and emotional side of living with diabetes. Social workers may be able to connect you with resources such as free medication programs for people who can't afford their drugs and free transportation to doctor's appointments. Psychologists and family counselors will be able to offer individual or family counseling to help you deal with the stress and depression that can sometimes accompany a chronic disease.

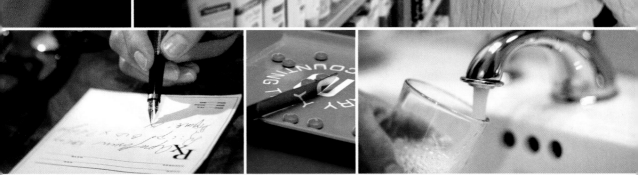

at the pharmacy

It's not just a place to pick up prescriptions; Come here for key supplies, expert advice, and answers about your medications—and ultimately, better control of your diabetes.

get friendly with the pharmacist

Until now, your only interaction with your pharmacist may have been from afar, watching him or her counting capsules or putting pills in bottles. But your pharmacist does far more than meets the eye (in fact, the person you see counting pills may be a technician and not the actual pharmacist). Your pharmacist can help you understand your diabetes medications, dispense advice, and even save you from dangerous drug interactions.

Shop at only one pharmacy. Having all your medication records in one place lessens your risk of taking duplicate medications (sometimes under different brand names) or experiencing dangerous drug interactions. You'll also feel more comfortable asking questions or bringing up concerns if you're friendly with your "drugstore doctor."

Check your prescription while you're at the store. Read the label and look at the pills or liquid as soon as you pick up your prescription, not when you get home, to make sure it's the right drug at the right dosage. If you're getting a medication you've taken before and it looks different, ask about it.

Ask to meet with your pharmacist to review your meds and get answers to questions you may have. Many pharmacies are creating designated areas or "education cubicles" where you can talk with a pharmacist.

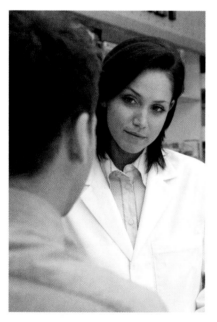

Call to schedule an appointment, and bring all your medications and any vitamins, herbal supplements, and other over-the-counter items you regularly take. It's possible that you are taking two medications that do the same thing, or two medications that counter each other—for example, one that lowers blood pressure and another that raises it. Before you leave the store, ask for a printout of your prescription medications for your records.

Take notes. Write down the answers to your questions or important points about new medications you're taking so you can review them at home, when you're under less pressure.

Have follow-up meetings with your pharmacist whenever you are changing, adding, or reducing medications.

Recruit your pharmacist's help to reduce medication costs. Ask her if she sees ways to reduce your pharmacy bill, perhaps by ordering 60-day supplies rather than 30-day supplies (you'll need the right prescription from your doctor to do this) or by taking an older or generic version of one or more of your medications, with your doctor's approval.

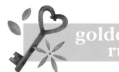

golden rule! Carry a List of All Medications and Supplements

This will be handy to have for visits with doctors, pharmacists, dietitians, and other health professionals. It could also prove helpful in the event of an emergency. Include supplements and over-the-counter remedies you regularly take. Next to the name of the medication or supplement, include the date of the prescription (where applicable), why you are taking the product (what is it supposed to do?), the dosage, and how many times a day you take it.

Never, ever go without your diabetes medications because you think you can't afford them. Many drug makers offer free medications for those who can't afford to buy them. Have your doctor or pharmacist contact the drug company to see if they have such a program and whether you qualify.

Disclose any allergies or adverse reactions to drugs. Make certain that allergic reactions or bad side-effects from any previous drugs are in your records. Be specific about your experience. Did you have a rash? Nausea? If you switch pharmacies, be sure to update your information.

Know who's who. Technicians help pharmacists by preparing medications, counting tablets, and labeling bottles. Pharmacy aides (the folks you usually see behind the counter) are often cashiers who primarily answer phones, handle money, and stock shelves. Neither is qualified to answer your medication questions, but they will pass along your questions to the pharmacist.

Ask about diabetes or other health test days. Many pharmacies are authorized to give flu shots and other vaccinations. Some larger drugstores also hold health days, or diabetes days, at which you can have your blood pressure, cholesterol, and A1C blood sugar tests done, as well as get a flu shot—all for an affordable fee. The visit usually includes face-to-face time with the pharmacist so you may be able to squeeze in a question or two.

See if your drug is available by mail order. Many insurance companies allow you to buy certain long-term medications in bulk, at cheaper prices, through the mail. Ask whether your drug in on the list.

Investigate online pharmacies. Comparison shopping at online pharmacies is a great way to find the best price for your medication. But be careful about which sites you use. The pharmacy should be approved by the National Association of Boards of Pharmacy. Go to www.nabp.org to see if it is. These pharmacies require you to fax or mail in your doctor's prescription. Never buy from a site that offers prescription drugs without prescriptions from your doctor, and only use an online pharmacy that offers access to a licensed pharmacist.

buying testing supplies

Having diabetes isn't quite like having, say, high cholesterol. There's simply more equipment involved. And be thankful it exists, because without blood-sugar meters, for instance, treating the disease would be like shooting in the dark. Now that there are more than 180 million people with diabetes in the world—and counting—it isn't surprising that many pharmacies are starting to dedicate special sections to diabetes supplies, or that you may need a little help wading through the options.

Before you buy supplies, find out which your insurance covers. Your pharmacy will have a variety of blood-glucose meters, test strips, lancets, and other supplies. But check with your insurance company before choosing. Most companies limit the types or brands you can buy for reimbursement or coverage.

Price test strips before you buy a meter. Over time you'll spend much more money on test strips than you will on a meter—strips are where manufacturers make their money. And not all strips can be used in all meters. So if your insurance company gives you a choice of which meters to buy, remember, the price of the strips is more important than the price of the meter. For the sake of convenience, be sure the meter's strips are carried by your pharmacy if you plan to buy them there.

Ask about meter options. If your insurance covers several types of meters, ask your doctor, your diabetes educator, and your pharmacist for suggestions. Also check the manufacturers' Web sites, where you'll find explanations of the different features, and sometimes, special offers. Again, your health plan will probably cover only certain test strips, which will limit your choice of meters. A great place to start your search for a blood

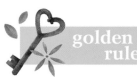

golden rule! **Test and Clean Your Meter Regularly**

If your monitor is old or dirty, if you've coded it improperly, or if your test strips have expired or been exposed to heat or dampness, you'll get incorrect readings, which are worse than useless—they're misleading. Be sure to follow the manufacturer's instructions for how and when to clean the machine. To make sure you're getting accurate readings from your meter, bring it to your doctor's appointment and use it to check your blood within a minute or two of when your doctor draws blood. According to the American Diabetes Association, the reading you get from your meter shouldn't be more than 15 percent off from what the lab analysis of your blood says.

glucose meter is in the annual resource guide put out by *Diabetes Forecast* magazine, published by the American Diabetes Association. It's available in many pharmacies, or you can see the 2007 version online at www.diabetes.org/diabetes-forecast/resource-guide.jsp. The guide doesn't recommend specific brands, but it gives a comprehensive outline of what is most current and available.

Figure out the features you want the most. Some meters require less blood than others and hold more readings than others. Some can talk you through the steps of taking and testing your blood. With others you can download results to your computer and even create charts to give you a picture of your glucose control at different times of the day over time. (If you buy this kind, make sure it will work with your home computer and your doctor's computer, too.) Work with your doctor or diabetes educator to figure out what features are most important for you. Some people like the bells and whistles; on the other hand, maybe a big display and ease of use are all you want.

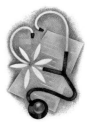

Heat and dampness can affect the shelf life of test strips.

Buy a meter that doesn't require coding. Since test strips may vary from batch to batch, some meters require you to enter a code (found on the vial of test strips). This calibrates the meter to the batch of test strips. Other models (those made by Bayer, for example) have a "no coding" feature. That's handy because forgetting to "code" a meter is cited as one of the most frequent reasons that blood glucose is recorded inaccurately.

Do the math to see if you can save money on test strips. If you don't have insurance that covers test strips, you might be able to lower your cost of strips and lancets (discussed on page 158) by buying bulk. (Health insurance providers won't pay for bulk items, so this tip applies only if your strips aren't paid for by insurance.) Do a quick calculation to see how many test strips you need. The strips have an expiration date, so you don't want to buy so many that you get stuck with out-of-date test strips. For example, if you test your blood sugar four times a day, you know you'll need around 120 a month.

Keep test strips cool and dry. The shelf life of test strips can be affected by heat and dampness. The bathroom is not a good place to store them.

Use the logbook that comes with your meter. The only way to know how various foods or exercise affects your blood sugar is to check your levels often and *write down the results.* Most meters include a notebook for this purpose; the pharmacy may also carry logbooks. Don't stop at recording your results; sit down and examine them, looking for patterns. Bring your logbook every time you visit your doctor, dietitian, and diabetes educator. They can help you make sense of the results.

Choose your own lancet. This is the little sharp tool that you'll use daily to puncture your finger. You'll see boxes of these along the shelves next to the blood-glucose meters. They come in varying widths and lengths. While you can use the lancet by itself, most people choose to use a lancing device, a gadget that spring-loads the lancet so you can quickly penetrate your skin. The quicker the penetration, the less the sting. Many glucose meters come with lancing devices, or even have them built in, but you are free to use a different lancet if you find one that works better for you. Your lancing device will last for a long time, but you'll have to stock plenty of lancets, which are designed for onetime use.

Buy a sharps container. These inexpensive puncture-proof containers have openings designed to let you drop used lancets, insulin syringes, and pen needles in without touching any of the unsanitary parts. They also lock when full for safety. Used strips, lancets, and syringes are considered biohazardous waste. Check with your local refuse department and ask how you should dispose of your container. You may be able to take your sharps containers to a local hospital, so call them and check.

Skip the alcohol pads. Before you prick your finger to check your blood sugar you do need to rid your hands of germs and oils that could throw off your meter's reading, but simply washing with soap and warm water will do the trick. Alcohol causes more of a sting when the lancet goes in (because the lancet brings some of the alcohol into the skin with it) and it also dries out your skin. If you do use alcohol, let it dry before pricking yourself.

stock up on other useful items

The wonders you can find in an average pharmacy! Nerve pain in your feet? There's a cream for that. Sunscreen? We'll tell you how to choose. Also discover an incredibly simple product to help you figure out if your weight is really a problem.

Buy a pill organizer. Many people who have diabetes take eight to 12 different medications, vitamins, and other supplements. Keeping track of that many pills is difficult, as is remembering which ones you have already taken, and what still needs to be swallowed. Pick up a pill organizer that has flip-top compartments to contain all your pills for each day of the week. You'll be able to tell at a glance which you have taken and which you have not.

Buy several bottles or gel packs of glucose. You'll see bottles of chewable tablets and gel tubes (they look like cake decorating tubes) on the shelves of the diabetes section of your drugstore. These products are made of glucose for treating low blood sugar. If you are particularly prone to low blood sugar episodes, it's a good idea to have several bottles or gel packs—one for the car, your desk at work, at home, and packed in your suitcase when traveling. Throw a few tablets into a zip-close bag to carry in your purse when you are heading out for an evening, a family picnic, or other outdoor event.

Keep feet happy with chafe-free socks. Pharmacies often carry socks for people with nerve damage or loss of sensation in their feet. These socks fit comfortably, but not too tight, and they don't have any seams that could cause sore spots or blisters. People with loss of sensation in their feet may not notice chafing from regular socks, and chafing could lead to blisters and infection.

Consider an at-home blood pressure monitor. If you struggle with high blood pressure, tracking your levels at home can help you keep track of your levels between doctor visits and maybe help you lower those levels. Home tests may even provide truer results than your doctor's test if you're one of those people who gets nervous in the doctor's office. Ask the pharmacist to tell you the cuff size you need for your arm. Your readings will be wrong if the cuff size is wrong. And make sure you can read the numbers on the monitor.

(continued on page 162)

herbs and supplements for diabetes

Can herbs or supplements help you control your diabetes? These 10 have shown some promise in lowering blood sugar, boosting insulin sensitivity, reducing high blood pressure and cholesterol, and more. Talk to you doctor before adding any new pill to your regimen, especially if it has the potential to lower your blood sugar. You may need to check your blood sugar more often and possibly have your doctor adjust your medication dosage. If you don't see results after a month or two, stop wasting your money.

1 | gymnema sylvestre

Main use: Lowering blood sugar

Typical dosage: 200 to 250 milligrams twice daily.

This plant's Hindi name translates as "sugar destroyer," and the plant is said to reduce the ability to detect sweetness. It's regarded as one of the most powerful herbs for blood-sugar control. It may work by boosting the activity of enzymes that help cells use glucose or by stimulating the production of insulin. Though it hasn't been studied extensively, it's not known to cause serious side effects.

2 | bitter melon

Main use: Lowering blood sugar

Typical dosage: 50 to 100 milliliters (approximately 3 to 6 tablespoons) of the juice daily.

The aptly named bitter melon is thought to help cells use glucose more effectively and block sugar absorption in the intestine. When Philippine researchers had men and women take bitter melon in capsule form for three months, they had slight, but consistently, lower blood sugar than those taking a placebo. Gastrointestinal problems are possible side effects.

3 | magnesium

Main use: Lowering blood sugar

Typical dosage: 250 to 350 milligrams once a day.

Magnesium deficiency is not uncommon in people with diabetes, and it can worsen high blood sugar and insulin resistance. Some studies suggest that supplementing with magnesium may improve insulin function and lower blood sugar levels, but other studies have shown no benefit. Have your doctor check you for deficiency before supplementing with magnesium.

4 | prickly pear cactus

Main use: Lowering blood sugar

Typical dosage: If you eat it as a food, aim for ½ cup of cooked cactus fruit a day. Otherwise, follow label directions.

The ripe fruit of this cactus has been shown in some small studies to lower blood sugar levels. You may be able to find the fruit in your grocery store, but if not, look for it as a juice or powder at health food stores. Researchers speculate that the fruit may possibly lower blood sugar because it contains components that work similarly to insulin. The fruit is also high in fiber.

5 | gamma-linolenic acid

Main use: Easing nerve pain

Typical dosage: 270 to 540 milligrams once a day.

Gamma-linolenic acid, or GLA, is a fatty acid found in evening primrose oil. Some research suggests that people with diabetes have lower than optimal levels of GLA, and studies have found that the supplement can reduce and prevent nerve pain associated with diabetes.

6 | chromium

Main use: Lowering blood sugar

Typical dosage: 200 micrograms once daily.

This trace mineral is thought to enhance the action of insulin as well as being involved in carbohydrate, fat, and protein metabolism. Some research shows that it helps normalize blood sugar—but only in people who are deficient in chromium.

7 | bilberry

Main use: Protecting the eyes and nerves

Typical dosage: 80 to 120 milligrams two times per day of standardized bilberry extract.

This relative of the blueberry contains powerful antioxidants in its fruit and leaves. These antioxidants, called anthocyanidins, seem to help prevent damage to tiny blood vessels that can result in nerve pain and retinopathy (damage to the eye's retina). Animal studies have also suggested that bilberry may lower blood sugar.

8 | alpha-lipoic acid

Main uses: Easing nerve pain, lowering blood sugar

Typical dosage: 600 to 800 milligrams a day.

Called ALA for short, this vitamin-like substance neutralizes many types of free radicals. A build-up of free radicals, caused in part by high blood sugar, can lead to nerve damage and other problems. ALA may also help muscle cells take up blood sugar. In a German study, a team of scientists had 40 adults take either an ALA supplement or a placebo. At the end of the four-week study, the ALA group had improved their insulin sensitivity 27 percent. The placebo group showed no improvement. Other studies have shown a decrease in nerve pain, numbness, and burning.

9 | fenugreek

Main use: Lowering blood sugar

Typical dosage: 5 to 30 grams with each meal or 15 to 90 grams with one meal per day.

These seeds, used in Indian cooking, have been found to lower blood sugar, increase insulin sensitivity, and reduce high cholesterol, according to several animal and human studies. The effect may be partly due to the seeds' high fiber content. The seeds also contain an amino acid that appears to boost the release of insulin. In one of the largest studies on fenugreek, 60 people who took 25 grams daily showed significant improvements in blood sugar control and post-meal spikes.

10 | ginseng

Main use: Lowering blood sugar

Typical dosage: 1 to 3 grams a day in capsule or tablet form, or 3 to 5 milliliters of tincture three times a day.

Known for its immune-boosting and disease-fighting benefits, this Chinese herb has several positive diabetes studies behind it. Researchers have found that ginseng slows carbohydrate absorption; increases cells' ability to use glucose; and increases insulin secretion from the pancreas. A team from the University of Toronto has repeatedly demonstrated that ginseng capsules lower blood glucose 15 to 20 percent compared to placebo pills.

161

Ask your doctor if you should check your cholesterol at home. Most drugstores now sell home cholesterol tests. Most are very accurate, if you use them properly (many require you to fast, which people tend to forget to do). They can be useful if you're taking a cholesterol-lowering drug and want to see how well it, and your dietary changes, are working between doctor visits. Look for a test that measures LDL ("bad") and HDL ("good") cholesterol in addition to total cholesterol. Some tests also measure triglycerides, blood fats associated with a higher risk of heart disease. Talk with your doctor about the results.

Stash a meal for on-the-go. Prepared snack bars and drinks for people with diabetes are big business. You may not need them at all ("real" foods are usually preferable). But if you're someone who's often caught without a snack at snack time or a meal at mealtime, you might want to keep a stash for emergencies. The carbohydrates they contain are digested slowly to help keep blood sugar levels steady.

Pick up a cloth measuring tape. This is one of the easiest ways to keep tabs on your heart health and to keep diabetes complications under control. Research shows that a waistline bigger than 35 inches for women and 40 for men is a red flag for increased risk of heart disease, high blood pressure, and stroke. You can also use the cloth tape to measure your ankles—if they are swollen it's a sign that you are retaining water, and your doctor should be notified. Water retention is a side effect of some diabetes drugs.

Buy—and use—a good moisturizer. High blood sugar can contribute to dry skin, which in turn can lead to cracks that can lead to infection—and then you're in trouble. So make a commitment to using moisturizer every day or night. While you'll see moisturizers labeled for people with diabetes, don't feel limited to these, which often cost more. Any moisturizer that's thick enough to stay put and that doesn't irritate your skin will do.

Forgo deodorant soaps. These tend to be drying and irritating to the skin, and dry, irritated skin is more likely to crack and become vulnerable to infection. Choose instead a moisturizing soap such as Dove.

For pain and tingling in your feet, buy a capsaicin cream. Capsaicin, a compound found in hot peppers, relieves pain over time by running interference between nerve cells and your brain. Give them a few weeks to work. And keep the creams away from your eyes, mouth, and nose—they can burn. Even thorough hand washing can leave capsaicin residue, which can sting if you touch your eyes, so it's a good idea to keep a pair of disposable gloves handy for applying the cream.

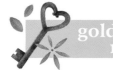

golden rule!   ## Set the Timer When You Brush Your Teeth

Dentists recommend brushing for two to three minutes to get teeth clean, but most of us spend far less time than that caring for our pearly whites. Set a timer and you'll realize just how long three minutes really is. Brushing thoroughly is especially important for people with diabetes, who are at increased risk for gum disease.

Choose sugar-free over-the-counter medicines when possible. Your blood sugar may already be on the high side when you're sick, so why get unnecessary sugar from cold and cough medicines? While the sugar in these won't affect your blood sugar much, neither will it hurt to look for sugar-free versions of cough syrups, lozenges, chewable aspirin, and decongestants in the diabetes aisle. If you don't see the items, ask your pharmacist where they are kept.

Buy the most protective sunscreen. Certain diabetes drugs and blood pressure drugs make the skin more sensitive to the sun, so it's especially important that you protect yourself. A bad sunburn can even raise your blood sugar and may take longer to heal than it would for someone else. Choose a sunscreen that has at least an SPF of 15 and look for a "broad-spectrum" brand that protects against both UVA and UVB light. These often contain ingredients such as Mexoryl, Helioplex, zinc oxide, or avobenzone (aka Parsol 1789).

Imagine a shot glass when you apply sunscreen. Experts say you need to use at least 2 tablespoons of sunscreen for your body to get adequate protection. That's about a shot-glass full. Most of us use far less. So slather it on! Apply it at least half an hour before heading out into the sun to give your skin a chance to absorb it, and reapply every two hours.

Throw out old sunscreen. If you've had a bottle that's been lying around for several years or has been living in the glove compartment of a hot car, buy a new bottle—yours has lost strength.

Replace your toothbrush every three months. If the bristles are frayed or bent outward, replace more frequently. Otherwise, your brush won't get your teeth as clean, and you'll be transferring tons of bacteria to your mouth. Look for a brush with soft bristles so you don't bruise your gums, and while you're in the toothbrush aisle, pick up some floss, too—then use it.

Consider an electric toothbrush. Studies show they do remove plaque better than manual brushes do.

how to choose vitamins and more

Most doctors recommend a daily multivitamin as cheap insurance on a healthy diet, but the shelves are lined with choices. Which do you pick? Do you need more than one vitamin supplement? Follow this advice, and be sure to check with your doctor before taking any new supplement.

Talk to your dietitian before buying. It's a good idea to discuss your vitamin needs with a registered dietitian or nutritionist. Once the specialist has a good idea of your eating habits and has run lab tests to check for deficiencies, he or she can make recommendations on what vitamins you'll need. You may be fine with a once-a-day vitamin, or your nutritionist may recommend some extra supplements based on your needs. Ask her to write down all recommendations and their dosage amounts.

Be wary of vitamin shop "experts." It's most likely that this person is not a registered dietitian or a certified health professional of any sort. Check any recommendations with your own registered dietitian before you buy.

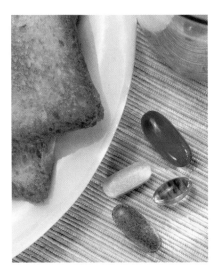

Check the Daily Values on your multi. While you'll try to get most of your nutrients from a healthy diet, a multivitamin is generally recommended as insurance for the nutrients we tend to fall short on. The Daily Values (DV) are a set of recommended nutrient amounts determined by the Food and Nutrition Board of the National Academy of Sciences and Health based on age and sex. Choose a multivitamin that says it contains 100 percent of the Daily Values of vitamins A, B_2, B_6, B_{12}, C, D, and E, along with folic acid, niacin, copper, and zinc.

Pick a high-potency multivitamin. This term indicates that a vitamin contains 100 percent of daily values for at least two-thirds of its listed nutrients. The rest you can get from eating nutritious meals that include lean protein, whole grains, and plenty of fresh fruits and vegetables.

Look for USP on the label. USP means that the product meets the voluntary standards of the U.S. Pharmacopoeia. Supplement companies can also voluntarily have their products tested through independent agencies.

Beware of other bells and whistles. Before you slap down your hard-earned cash for a formula that promises better immune health or boasts super-high levels of antioxidants, discuss the best options for you with your registered dietitian. It's probably better to focus on eating a diet full of vegetables and fruits than to seek a few extra ingredients in a multi.

Take your vitamins with a meal. Some vitamins and supplements can cause nausea if taken on an empty stomach, so plan on taking your pills with a meal. Some people find it easier to remember their vitamins if they get in the habit of taking their supplements routinely with breakfast, lunch, or dinner.

Ask your doctor about iron. Many multis contain iron, but men and post-menopausal women don't usually need more of this mineral beyond what they get from food, so ask your doctor if you should choose a multi that does or doesn't contain it. Too much iron can cause toxic effects. If you are concerned that your iron levels may be low (for instance, if you are a strict vegetarian), ask your doctor to check your iron levels with a blood test.

If you're a woman, take calcium supplements. A lack of calcium and vitamin D (see tip below) has been strongly linked to an increased risk of developing diabetes. If you already have diabetes, these supplements can still do you good by protecting your bones—especially important since older folks with diabetes are more prone to osteoporosis and bone fractures than their counterparts who don't have diabetes. Calcium also helps your body with contractions of muscles and blood vessels. Take 1,000 milligrams a day, or 1,200 milligrams a day if you're a women over 50. Take it in split doses of 500 or 600 milligrams in the morning and evening; the body can't absorb higher doses. Men should check with their doctors before supplementing with calcium.

Should You Take Antioxidants?

It's a good question. It seems that people with diabetes do need more of certain antioxidants, such as vitamins C and E, and that antioxidants play a role in preventing diabetes complications such as nerve damage and eye problems. One study even found that supplementing with vitamin E (400 IU), vitamin C (500 to 1,000 milligrams), magnesium (300 to 600 milligrams), and zinc (30 milligrams) daily for three months significantly lowered blood sugar in a test group. But other studies on antioxidant supplements have yielded mixed results, and supplements aren't without dangers. Too much magnesium, for instance, can potentially be harmful in people with decreased kidney function. And a study that looked at the mineral selenium and its affect on skin cancer revealed that the supplement increased the risk of diabetes by nearly 50 percent.

Much more research is under way, but for now, most experts advise getting the bulk of your antioxidants from a diet rich in fruits, vegetables, and beans, and filling any gaps with a basic multivitamin.

Take a Daily Low-Dose Aspirin

According to the American Diabetes Association, people with diabetes have a two- to fourfold chance of dying from heart disease. Since studies show that taking a daily low-dose aspirin (83 milligrams, also known as a "baby aspirin") can cut your risk of heart attack by as much as 60 percent, the association currently recommends that people with diabetes take a low-dose aspirin daily, unless you are allergic to aspirin. Check with your doctor first, of course.

Make sure your calcium supplements also contain vitamin D. Experts are learning more and more about the important roles vitamin D plays in the body. For instance, low levels are associated with increased insulin resistance and decreased insulin secretion. Obese people are at higher risk for D deficiency, and D deficiency seems to predispose people to become obese. D is also emerging as an important anticancer vitamin. Make sure your calcium pill contains at least 200 IU of vitamin D, which also helps the body use the calcium in the pill.

Ask your doctor about fish oil capsules. Many studies show that taking fish oil can lower the risk of heart attack and stroke risk by lowering LDL ("bad") cholesterol and triglyceride levels, helping to prevent dangerous blood clots and more. That's good news for people with diabetes, who are at an increased risk for both conditions. Fish oil also combats low-grade inflammation in the body, which contributes to diabetes and other chronic diseases. But fish oil supplements aren't for everyone, so ask for your doctor's advice. Taking the supplements with food can help reduce the burping often associated with fish oils, as can choosing a fish-oil supplement that contains citrus essence. A typical dosage is 1 to 3 grams daily.

chapter ten

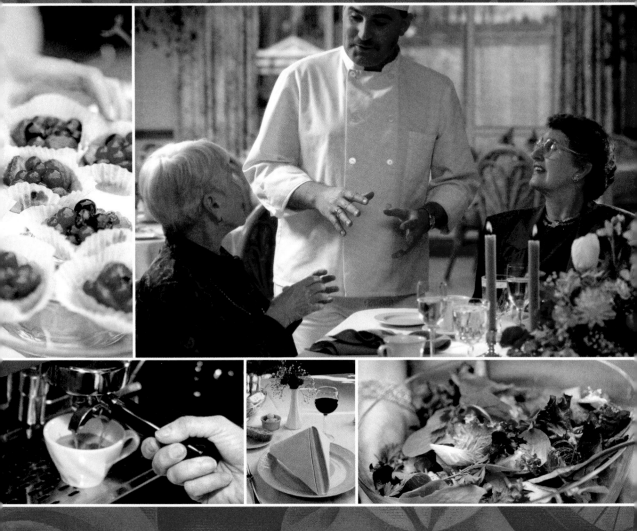

at a restaurant

Who doesn't love dining out? When you eat out, eat smart—
just as you would at home—and the price you pay will be
the check, not your health.

get set before you sit down

Low lighting, soft music, indulgent wait staff, mouthwatering scents wafting from the kitchen: Restaurants are in the business of making you feel like a VIP, because the longer you stay and the more devil-may-care your attitude about how much you eat and how much you spend, the more money the restaurant makes. The best way not to overindulge your stomach or your wallet is to step through the door prepared.

Sneak an advance peek at the menu. The best way not to let the atmosphere dissolve your determination to eat well is to do a little reconnaissance work before you even leave the house. Look online for the menus of chain restaurants and some upper-tier restaurants; some chains even post nutritional information. Look for options that fit into your eating plan—and identify those that you promise yourself you'll stay away from.

Scan the menu for a "special diet" section. Many people these days are trying to make healthy choices when they dine out, and restaurants are taking notice. Most eateries have a list of no-frills healthy dishes on their menus; most meats are baked or braised, and vegetables are usually steamed. If you're really counting calories and fat grams, head straight for this section of the menu.

Never "save up" calories. If you're tempted to skimp on breakfast or lunch so you can indulge in a bigger dinner, resist. For anyone with diabetes, it's important to eat the same amounts of food at about the same

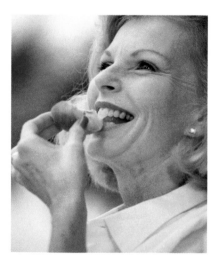

time of day every day to help ensure steady blood sugar. And skipping lunch before a big dinner out could very well backfire—you'll find it nearly impossible to resist the bread on the table when you walk in, and defenses against fatty, high-calorie main dishes will be down.

Have a healthy snack at home an hour before your restaurant reservation. That's assuming that you're eating an hour later than you normally do, as people tend to do when they eat out. (If you're eating at the normal time and you didn't have an afternoon snack planned, skip it.) Munch on a small piece of fruit and an ounce of low-fat string cheese, or a couple of pieces of celery slathered with a tablespoon of peanut or almond butter.

Not only will a snack curb your appetite, but the feeling of having just eaten will keep you from mindlessly picking at the complimentary bread or tortilla chips.

whip it together! Ambrosia

This treat, under 150 calories, tastes best after it's chilled in the fridge for a few hours, making it the perfect "nightcap" dessert after a dinner out.

Cut a small **pineapple** into 1-inch chunks (or use about a cup of canned fruit) and slice 2 large **bananas** ¼-inch thick. Toss both into a nonreactive bowl. Peel and section three **navel oranges** over the bowl, allowing the juice from the oranges to coat the fruit. Gently fold in ½ cup miniature **marshmallows** and 2 tablespoons sweetened flaked **coconut**. Cover with plastic wrap and refrigerate for at least 2 hours. Before serving, garnish with fresh **mint** sprigs. Serves 6.

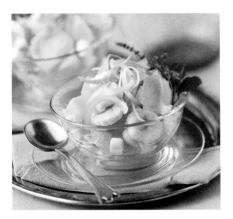

Before you go out, prepare a healthy, homemade dessert. Prepare a light berry crumble, a sugar-free gelatin with fresh fruit, or a baked apple sprinkled with cinnamon and sugar substitute. Later, when you're at the restaurant and you're handed the dessert menu—or even worse, when a waiter brings over a tray filled with fatty, sugary confections—you'll remember that you have a treat waiting for you at home.

Wear a fancy blouse and/or close-fitting pants. Whether you dine at a four-star eatery or a diner, what you wear can affect what your order. With tight pants tugging at your tummy, you literally won't have room to gorge on a big dinner. And chances are, if you are wearing your favorite blouse, you'll be afraid of ruining it, and you'll shy away from heavily sauced or oily entrées. The worst thing to wear? Stretchy or elastic-waist pants with room for expansion.

In the parking lot, pop a piece of gum into your mouth. Just as brushing your teeth early in the evening keeps you from late-night snacking, popping a fresh piece of mint chewing gum just before you go into the restaurant will help you pass up sugary sodas and other predinner temptations. Only after the waiter takes your order should you discreetly toss out the gum; that still gives you at least 15 minutes or so for your mouth to return to normal and your dinner entrée to taste as enjoyable as you'd hoped.

smart dining-out strategies

A generation ago, restaurant meals were reserved for special occasions. Now we eat out so often that we don't even bother to get dressed up—and sometimes, we even opt for takeout because we can't be bothered to sit down and be served! Why not take a page from the past, and inject a little excitement and eventfulness back into your restaurant outings? Whether you realize it or not, little decisions like where you should dine, with whom you eat, and what you do after you dine can all help you control your diabetes.

Splurge on an upscale restaurant. Look for a restaurant that prides itself on using in-season, local ingredients. Such places tend to serve smaller portions of really top-quality foods, rather than gargantuan platters of inexpensive oily pastas and pizzas. How do you know if the ingredients are local? The menu will usually say where top-quality fish, meat, or produce is from. If a chef has gone through the trouble and expense of acquiring, say, fresh wild salmon from a local river, he'll want you to know how special it is and will want to prepare the fish in a way that will show its quality to best advantage. This means that the chef probably won't fry it or hide it under heavy sauces—fewer grams of fat and calories for you.

Dine with other health-conscious people. Research shows that diners tend to mimic the people around them. That means that if your friends order grilled fish and salads with the dressing on the side, you're more likely to do so, too. Sample all of the entrées when they're served. The variety will make you feel like you indulged more than you really did—and you'll know what you want to order next time.

Frequent the same restaurants over and over. If you dine out often, this advice is for you. The more new choices you're faced with, the more easily you'll be seduced by foods you probably shouldn't be eating. Limit temptation by ordering from the same old menu and choosing dishes you know work well for your blood sugar.

Plan an all-out sinful meal out twice a year. You've been dreaming of that triple brownie sundae and homemade pasta at the local Italian restaurant since your last anniversary dinner there. So go! Always saying "no" to food treats can make you resent your healthy diet. And even nutritionists say that they go out and have their "weakness" food—maybe it's onion rings, French fries, or ice cream—once every six or eight months. To get maximum enjoyment out of your special meal, make a reservation a month or two in advance. The farther in advance your event is planned, the more pleasure you'll get when you finally dig in.

golden rule!   Save Restaurant Meals for Special Occasions

Several studies have found that the more people eat out, the more likely they are to be obese, and extra weight can make your insulin resistance worse—and your blood sugar harder to control. In one study, researchers followed more than 3,000 adults for 15 years, keeping track of their body weight, changes in insulin resistance, and how often they ate at fast-food restaurants. They found that people who ate fast food more than twice a week gained an average of 10 more pounds over 15 years than people who ate fast food less than once a week. Frequent fast-food eaters also had double the risk of becoming insulin resistant.

Ask the waiter to "recork" your wine. Ordering wine by the bottle is usually a better deal than buying it by the glass (unless there are only two of you and you're sure you're each going to drink only one glass). But don't have seconds just to finish the bottle. Ask the waiter to put the cork back in, and take the rest of the bottle home. In the United States, this is perfectly legal in most states, even if the restaurant doesn't exactly advertise the option.

Save the gossip for your post-meal walk. Even a casual lunch with an old friend can turn into an exercise opportunity if you take an energized turn or two around a nearby park or the mall afterward. Light exercise is a sure way to help level your blood sugar if a meal has caused it to spike.

Check your blood sugar two hours after your meal. If the result is within your target range, you'll know to order the same thing when you go back. If it's not, avoid those dishes next time, or try making adjustments to your meal, such as declining the bread or substituting a vegetable for the rice or potato.

Invite your group out for frozen yogurt after dinner. Sheer inertia and sluggishness after a filling restaurant meal can cause you to order a dessert that you didn't really want—and finish the whole thing. That can ruin a carefully chosen meal, considering that a single slice of cheesecake contains about 720 calories and 25 grams of saturated fat. If you don't have a healthy dessert at home that's ready to eat, walk to the nearest place that serves frozen yogurt. And who knows? You might even decide on the way over that you're too full for dessert after all.

at the table

Ever go to a party determined to have a good time? Well, when you sit down at a restaurant table, be equally determined to eat well—and have fun. Focus on soaking in the atmosphere and enjoying the time with your spouse and friends, and yes, the food, in moderation.

Ask the waiter not to bring bread. You're likely to get plenty of starch in your meal (from your rice, potato, and starchy vegetables such as corn), so save your carbohydrates for later.

After you're seated, take a quick stroll around the dining room. Before you place your order, excuse yourself to wash your hands, and take the long route to the restroom. On your way there, get a good look at other diners' dishes. This reconnaissance mission can be a bigger help in deciding what to order than the most well-meaning waiter. You'll see how big the portions are, if tonight's specials look good, and whether the vegetable sides are bathed in butter. When you return to your seat, you'll be the most well-informed diner in the room.

Order a garden salad to start. A small garden salad contains at least two servings of vegetables and about 5 grams of fiber. Because of that fiber, salads are surprisingly filling. In fact, a study published in the *Journal of the American Dietetic Association* found that women who ate 100-calorie salads before their entrées consumed about 12 percent fewer calories during the meal. Just stick to veggies in the salad, rather than fatty meats, cheeses, and nuts.

Dress your own salad, rather than letting the chef do it for you. It's true: A tasty dressing can absolutely make a salad. The problem is, chefs know this, too, and can be heavy-handed when tossing the dressing in the salad. A typical restaurant Caesar salad is tossed with 2½ ounces of dressing, which adds about 360 calories and 38 grams of fat to otherwise

golden rule! Eat Only as Much as You Would at Home

It's not at all unusual for a restaurant meal to contain more than half a day's worth of calories and fat. Eating a mega-size portion can not only wreak havoc with your blood sugar, it could cause you to overeat for the next two days. When researchers studied the eating habits of 32 people, they found that when the subjects ate 50 percent more at a meal, they continued to eat 16 percent more calories for two days than when they ate a normal-sized meal. When their portion sizes doubled, they ate 26 percent more calories for two days.

healthy and very low-cal Romaine lettuce. Ordering the same dressing on the side and topping your salad with just a tablespoon would add 77 calories and 8 grams of fat to your greens.

Alternatively, start your meal with a clear soup. This is another proven strategy to take the edge off your hunger and help you eat less of the main meal. In one Penn State University study, people who ate a broth-based vegetable soup before lunch ended up consuming, on average, 20 percent fewer calories overall. Avoid cheesy or creamy soups, such as French onion, baked potato, and broccoli-cheese.

Think for yourself when you order. Some restaurants hire consultants to tell them where to put what on the menu and how to price it—and it's money, not health, that they're after. For instance, they'll typically place dishes that they want you to buy just above the center of the menu's first right-hand page. The two top and bottom dishes on a list are also the ones that diners remember most, so restaurant owners tend to put their most expensive items in those places. The specialties (which also tend to be more expensive) might appear in big type, and cheaper meals in small type.

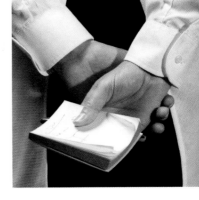

Speak up and ask for small changes to your dish. Don't be shy; most restaurants are happy to oblige, within reason. Just make your requests simple. If the item you have your eye on is fried, ask if it can be grilled instead. If it's coated in a buttery sauce, ask if the sauce can be left off. And remember that chefs aren't miracle workers. If you're tempted to make an unreasonable request, like asking for macaroni and cheese without the cheese, order something else.

Befriend the wait staff. If your server has gone out of her way to ask the chef to broil your meat, steam your vegetables, and put your sauce on the side, make a point of learning her name, thanking her, and leaving a generous tip. The next time you're in the restaurant, ask to be seated in her section. She'll eventually automatically do the things that you always ask her to do, like bringing you one piece of bread—whole wheat. Restaurant regulars who are kind and generous to servers are always taken care of. (Waiters talk about your generosity, too, so you're bound to get good service even if you're seated in another section.)

Have an appetizer and a salad instead of an entrée. Many restaurants' entrées are at least twice as big as a standard serving. If you don't think you have the willpower to order a main course and *not* eat the whole thing, order an appetizer-size dish instead. Healthy options include shrimp cocktail, steamed mussels, hummus and pita bread, and grilled chicken skewers (with sauce on the side). Ask the server to bring you one of these as your entrée, and dig into a salad when everyone else is eating their deep-fried appetizers. You'll still enjoy two courses—you've just made smarter choices.

Substitute a side of broccoli for your French fries. Want to order the turkey burger platter but don't want to be tempted by the French fries? Ask to substitute the restaurant's vegetable of the day for the fries. A half cup of cooked broccoli, for example, contains no fat and just 27 calories— less than one-tenth the calories in a small order of French fries! Making the easy switch from fries to broccoli also saves you 3 grams of saturated fat and infuses your meal with about 80 percent of your daily allowance of vitamin C.

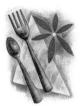

Cream- or cheese-based sauces can double the number of calories in a dish.

Skip the buffet. If the restaurant boasts all-you-can-eat shrimp platters and bottomless buffets, steer clear, no matter how great the price. One research study found that when people served themselves food, as they do at buffets, they often gave themselves over 25 percent more food than a healthy portion. All-you-can-eat platters are just as bad—maybe worse—because the plate portion may look reasonable, but you quickly lose count of how many full plates you've been served.

Fix your gaze on a visual reminder. Creamed spinach, mashed potatoes, and chicken-fried steak sound mighty good, but there's more saturated fat on that plate than you should eat in two days. It's moments like this when you'll be glad that you have a secret weapon in your purse or pocket. Perhaps it's a photo of you a few years ago, looking very happy and 20 pounds lighter. Maybe it's a photograph of a lost relative who had diabetes and didn't take care of it well enough. Your visual aid might even be a list of health goals you want to accomplish—anything that will nudge you to make a healthier choice.

Forgo "smothered" food and heavy sauces. "Smothered" usually means that a meat is bathed in a cream- or cheese-based sauce. This can double the number of calories in the dish, not to mention adding artery-clogging saturated fat. A standard serving of fettuccine Alfredo contains about 25 grams of saturated fat—more than the 15 grams a heart-healthy 2,000-calorie diet allows in an entire day. Bearing in mind that restaurants' portions can be double or triple a normal "serving," you could be consuming four to six times your daily allowance of saturated fat in one sitting.

Learn restaurant code words for "very high in fat." It's a common trend today for restaurants to make their food sound fancier and healthier than

golden rule! ## Order Your Meat or Fish Grilled, Baked, or Broiled

Dishes that are grilled, broiled, or baked will almost always be lower in fat than those that are fried or sautéed. An order of fried chicken tenders can contain as many as 23 grams of saturated fat, while a piece of grilled chicken or fish may only have 2 or 3 grams. Keeping your intake of saturated fat low—those following a 2,000-calorie diet should eat a maximum of 15 grams of saturated fat per day—is crucial for people with diabetes. Saturated fat contributes to insulin resistance, which makes controlling your blood sugar more difficult; saturated fat also increases your risk for heart disease.

it is. One of the biggest tricks they'll pull on customers is to disguise dishes that are deep-fried: Anything that's called "golden," "crispy," or—our favorite—"hand-battered" is deep-fried and should be avoided. Other words to look out for include "au gratin," "cheesy," "creamy," "buttered," and "béarnaise," all of which mean tons of cheese, cream, and/or butter.

Look for dishes that are poached or braised rather than sautéed. Technically speaking, sautéed foods should be cooked on high heat with a *small* amount of fat, but restaurants are heavy-handed with butter and oil because they make food taste better, says Robyn Golberg, RD, a nutritionist in Beverly Hills, California. Tossing in an extra spoonful of oil can add as many as 11 grams of fat to your meal. Instead, ask for dishes in which your meat is cooked in broth or wine, with minimal added fats. (The wine will burn off during cooking while the flavor remains.)

Ask for your vegetables steamed, not sautéed. Like sautéed entrées, sautéed veggies are often coated with more butter or oil than you need.

Order "blackened" or "Cajun" chicken or fish. "Blackened" means that the meat has been coated in Cajun seasoning and thrown into a red-hot cast-iron skillet. Cajun seasoning blends cayenne pepper, black pepper, and onion and garlic powders, so it delivers a little kick. It's a great way to get big flavor without sauces, oils, or other added calories.

Splurge on the lobster tail, but nix the melted butter. A 6-ounce lobster tail isn't unhealthy: It contains only a few grams of fat, 5 grams of carbs, and 200 calories. The real danger lies in the dish of melted butter that comes along with the crustacean. The simple act of squeezing lemon juice on your lobster rather than drowning it in 4 tablespoons of melted butter will save you an incredible 400 calories—probably about the same number of calories you eat for lunch!—and 28 grams of saturated fat.

controlling your portion size

The restaurant business is highly competitive; about 60 percent of restaurants fail within their first three years. So they have to find a way to get you in and keep you coming back. As one restaurant consultant Thomas J. Haas puts it, "The customer's perception of value should always come first"—and what most diners perceive as "good value" is a lot of food for not a lot of money. If you rid yourself of that notion, your body will go home happy.

Split an entrée. Most meals are large enough to split, so do it! Just order an extra side salad and extra vegetable if you like. You'll save tons of money, too.

Look for words like "queen," "junior," "senior," and "half-portion" on the menu. A "queen" or "junior" cut of prime rib, for example, is about 4 ounces less beef than a full cut. "Half-portions" are smaller-size versions of very filling entrées (like pastas or rice dishes) and are usually eaten as appetizers. Dishes on "senior" menus are meant for senior citizens and are priced at a discount but are also usually smaller than full-sized portions.

At steakhouses, order by weight. Unlike just about any other type of restaurant, steakhouses are specific about the weight, in ounces, of their portions—you can get the 8-ounce filet, or the 12-ounce sirloin, for example. This is both good news and bad for people watching their portion sizes: Good news because you know how much meat you're getting, but bad news because even the smallest portion will be bigger than the recommended 3 or 4 ounces. Pick the smallest boneless (so the weight of the bone is not factored in) steak on the menu, and ask that a portion of it be wrapped up immediately.

Visualize proper portion sizes and compare them to what's on your plate. If you've practiced portion control at home, it should be just as easy to do at a restaurant. A serving of meat (about 3 ounces) should be the size of a deck of cards, and a serving of pasta is half a cup (about half the size of a baseball) if you're having it as a side dish and twice that if it's your main course. If your entrée arrives and your meat takes up half the plate, you'll know to cut it in half and take the rest home or give it to a friend who's dining with you.

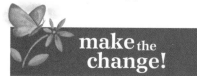

make the change!

The habit: Asking the waiter to put half your meal in a doggie bag before he serves it.

The result: You'll eat half the calories.

The proof: Several studies have shown that the more food is on the plate, the more people will eat. In one study by Cornell University, students served themselves at a buffet, and researchers measured how much they ate. A week later, the same students returned and were served either 100 percent, 125 percent, or 150 percent of the amount of the same meal. The students ate significantly more when they were given more food, even though they were told that they didn't have to eat everything on their plates. Another survey by the American Institute for Cancer Research found that seven out of 10 people clear their plates when they're at a restaurant.

Order tomorrow's lunch tonight. If you are dining at a restaurant famous for its generous portions and you know before you sit down that you'll be leaving with a doggie bag, start thinking before you order about which dishes will taste best tomorrow. Seafood and foods with thick, creamy sauces generally don't keep well, but steak, pork loin, chicken breast, and carved turkey all do—they can even be better the second day! The more vividly you can picture yourself digging in to a delicious steak sandwich tomorrow afternoon, the more likely you'll be not to gorge yourself on a gigantic dinner tonight.

Be on your best behavior, and you'll eat less. Whether you're dining at a casual family eatery or a four-star restaurant, you can actually consume less if you're perfectly behaved. For example, wait until everyone in your party has arrived, ordered, and received their food to dig in to your appetizers. Keep your mouth busy by making polite conversation with everyone at the table, rather than stuffing your face while you listen in. Put your fork down after every bite or two, and dab your lips with a napkin, or take a sip of water. Chew your food thoroughly before speaking. See how good behavior can actually slow your eating?

Stay away from your "downfall" foods. You know your weaknesses. If you can't possibly stop at a half cup of pasta, don't think about ordering it. If you tend to go overboard on the meat, order a big salad or fish. In a two-week study of 48 women with a history of binging, researchers found that half of their binges occurred in restaurants, nearly half happened at dinner, and more than half occurred on the weekends. Common binge foods included bread or pasta, sweets, high-fat meat, and salty snacks.

Leave three bites of food on your plate. If you're in the habit of clearing your plate at every meal only to feel indigestion later on, you're learning the hard way that it takes 20 or 30 minutes for your brain to register that you're 100 percent satiated. How much you can eat and feel pleasingly satisfied varies by individual; tonight, leave a few bites on your plate and see how you feel after your meal. Still stuffed? Tomorrow night leave a few more bites on the plate, and so on, until you're not feeling sick and sluggish after dinner.

Ask for extra napkins. Place the napkins over the plate if you don't want to eat any more food.

If you order dessert, order only one for the table. Ask for spoons or forks for everyone. One bite that you savor can satisfy your craving and save you lots of calories and carbs.

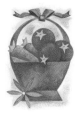

If you tend to go overboard on the meat, order a big salad or fish.

drinking and dining

Alcohol has different effects on people with diabetes than it does on other people. It can cause low blood sugar for one thing. The good news is that light to moderate alcohol intake (a maximum of one serving for women and two for men per day) is associated with a lower risk of dying of heart disease. Follow these guidelines, and a mug of beer or a glass of wine can be part of your dining experience.

Have a glass of wine or beer only if your blood sugar typically falls within your target range. If you check your blood sugar regularly, experts say that it's fine for both men and women to order up to two drinks at dinner. But if your levels are more erratic, take a pass—alcohol could cause you to experience hypoglycemia and will make it more difficult for you to get your blood sugar into your target range.

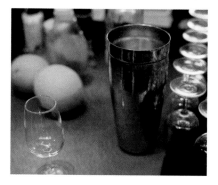

Ask the waiter to serve your cocktail with your meal. Having it before dinner is not a good idea, particularly for those who take insulin or other diabetes medications. Without food in your stomach, your blood sugar levels are likely already low. Drink your alcohol with food—or better yet, at the end of the meal—to lessen your chances of developing hypoglycemia.

Skip the "umbrella" drinks. Fancy cocktails with umbrellas contain a lot more sugar and calories than other cocktails do. A frozen piña colada, for example, packs 250 calories, 6 grams of fat, and 32 grams of carbs. A 1.5-ounce shot of whiskey mixed in with club seltzer or diet soda contains about 100 calories and no carbohydrates.

Decide whether you want wine or dessert. It's easy to forget that beverages contain calories, just as solid foods do. If your blood sugar levels are within a healthy range, it's fine to indulge in a glass of wine with dinner, but you'll need to modify your food intake. A 5-ounce glass of wine contains about 120 calories, for example—two glasses contain roughly the same amount of calories as a 2-square-inch brownie. If you're counting calories, you'll need to plan ahead and decide whether a drink or a sweet treat is more appealing. If you are on insulin, you can't substitute alcohol for the carb-filled dessert. Your insulin dose is based on the amount of carbs you eat. Alcohol has calories but you don't need insulin to cover it.

Don't confuse low blood sugar with inebriation. Sometimes slurred speech or difficulty speaking occurs with hypoglycemia; this could be confused with inebriation.

using your noodle at Chinese and Thai eateries

The good news about dining out at Chinese and Thai restaurants is that both cultures' foods really allow vegetables to shine—you're more likely to find a wide array of vegetarian dishes at these eateries than you are at almost any other type of restaurant. Protein-rich tofu, too, is plentiful; butter and cream sauces are almost unheard of. The bad news is that Chinese and Thai dishes can be clogged with sodium, sugar, and calorie-heavy oils; it's not uncommon for a single Chinese dish to contain an entire day's worth of sodium. And just half a cup of the coconut milk in Thailand's zesty curries contains more than a day's worth of saturated fat.

Fill your teacup. Whether the restaurant serves green or black tea, have some. Tea is one of nature's most powerful sources of antioxidants, and these free-radical scavengers help protect the body from the ravages of blood sugar, such as artery and nerve damage. Best of all, tea is calorie free.

Eat with chopsticks. It's easy to shovel big mouthfuls of food in with a fork. With chopsticks, each vegetable, grain of rice, or slice of beef has to be picked up carefully and delivered safely into your mouth. Because of the skill and pace involved, odds are, you'll eat more slowly with chopsticks than you will with a fork. And when you eat with chopsticks, you're more likely to leave some of the fatty sauce behind on the plate.

Avoid sweet-and-sour sauces. These sauces, which often come with lemon chicken or crispy orange beef, spell double trouble for the Chinese restaurant diner: Not only are they high in sugar, but they also traditionally coat meats that have been battered and deep fried.

Order garlic or brown sauce, on the side. These contain less sugar than sweet-and-sour sauces, and they often come with sautéed meat and vegetable dishes. They're typically sky-high in sodium, though, so ask for them on the side and use sparingly.

Order shrimp rather than beef. When the Center for Science in the Public Interest conducted a nutritional analysis of Chinese food, they found that some of the healthiest choices (in terms of fat and calorie content) were shrimp dishes, such as Szechuan shrimp and shrimp with garlic sauce. You still need to ask for the sauce on the side, to keep the sodium down.

Limit yourself to a few spoonfuls of brown rice. Let the others at the table help themselves to rice while you focus on the vegetables and protein in the meal. One-third cup of rice (one diabetic exchange, if you're using the exchange system) raises your blood sugar at the same rate as one slice of bread. You probably wouldn't think of eating six slices of bread during dinner, but you can easily load up on two cups of rice. Stick to ⅓ cup, and choose brown over white for extra fiber.

Order entrées that contain at least one green vegetable—or go vegetarian. Try spinach with garlic, beef and broccoli, or chicken with mixed vegetables. Avoid eggplant, which soaks up oil like a sponge. One eggplant in garlic sauce dish can contain an amazing 1,000 calories.

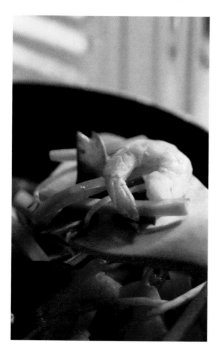

Order one vegetable dish and one other entrée and split them both. If you're dining with a friend, this strategy will give you more vegetables and more variety. Thai food in particular includes a wonderful selection of vegetables, such as bean sprouts, mushrooms, green and red chilies, and snow peas, along with fresh herbs such as lemongrass and basil.

Ask for less oil. Even a plate of stir-fried vegetables contains approximately 500 calories thanks to all the oil the restaurant uses. Ask them to use less, and they'll usually oblige.

Choose your Thai soup carefully. Thai restaurants offer tom yum goong (hot and sour soup), as well as vegetable and tofu soups made with clear broth. They're much better bets than soups like tom kha gai (chicken and lemongrass soup made with fatty coconut milk).

Order steamed pork dumplings or spring rolls rather than egg rolls—and plan to share. The dumplings are a reasonable 80 calories each (limit yourself to one or two), and spring rolls (which are similar to egg rolls, except that they're steamed instead of deep fried) are only about 100 calories each (limit yourself to one). They're both better choices than egg rolls, which have about 200 calories and 6 grams of saturated fat each.

Say no to the barbecued spare ribs. With 600 calories and 14 grams of saturated fat for four ribs, there's no less healthy appetizer at a Chinese restaurant. Choose the steamed pork or veggie dumplings instead.

Bring a big party of friends and eat your meal "family style." Here's a great strategy if you love Chinese or Thai food but just don't have the willpower to take home half your meal: Go out with five friends, and order just three or four main courses. With everyone filling up on rice (you should go easy on it), hot tea, and maybe an appetizer for the table, you'll have more than enough food for six people. Not only is this is a great way to sample a variety of dishes on the menu, it's easier to say no to rice if you have a variety of meats and veggies on the plate in front of you.

Never add soy sauce or duck sauce. Because your meal likely already contains a day's worth of sodium or more, resist the temptation to add the duck, hot mustard, hoisin, and soy sauces the restaurant provides. Just a tablespoon of regular soy sauce will add an extra 1,000 milligrams of sodium to your meal—half of the recommended daily maximum. A tablespoon of hoisin sauce has 250 milligrams of sodium, while duck sauce and hot mustard have 100 milligrams per tablespoon.

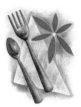

Keep your rice away from the fatty sauce on your plate.

Keep your entrée and rice in separate bowls. The surest path to maximum calorie intake at a Chinese restaurant is to scoop white rice onto your plate and dump your sauce-laden entrée on top. The rice will soak up the sauce, which will make you want to eat every last bite of it. Instead, do as the Chinese do and keep your rice in your rice bowl, and your meat and vegetables in the bowl it came in. Using your chopsticks to first pick up a slice of meat, and then perhaps a few grains of rice from the other bowl, accomplishes two things: You leave the fatty sauce behind on the plate, and you eat less rice.

Avoid coconut milk at all costs. Some of the best Thai dishes are the spicy, coconut milk-based curries, like green and massaman curry. As delicious as they are, they contain one of the most fattening ingredients imaginable: coconut milk. From just 1 ounce of coconut milk, you'd get 6 grams of fat, 5 of which are saturated. And you can be sure that any Thai curry or soup that contains coconut milk contains more than an ounce. Opt instead for jungle curry, which typically doesn't contain coconut milk, or dishes with a garlic-based sauce.

Order tofu steamed, not deep fried. Tofu is a popular ingredient in many Asian cuisines. It's an excellent protein source, packing about 2 grams per ounce, and contains only 183 calories. Try it instead of chicken, beef, or pork the next time you're at a Chinese or Thai restaurant. Just be sure to order it steamed or sautéed, not deep fried, or you'll cancel out the benefits.

Skip noodle-based dishes like pad Thai and Chinese lo mein. Though the classic Thai dish is one of the most popular and delicious, it's extremely high in calories and fat. A dish of beef pad Thai contains more than 1,300 calories, an unbelievable 60 grams of fat, and 126 grams of carbs. An order of Chinese house lo mein is similarly high in calories—it contains about 960—and has over 3,400 grams of sodium. That's about as much salt as you should eat over the course of two entire days.

when Mexican is on the menu

Despite the deep-fried, crispy tortilla chips and the prevalence of sour cream and cheese as toppings, Mexican food can be quite healthy if you know what to order. Fresh salsa, for example, contains just 10 calories a tablespoon, and black—not refried—beans are chock full of fiber. Here's how to build a better Mexican meal so you can have the "whole enchilada" with less fat and fewer calories.

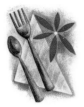

A deep-fried taco shell adds nearly 500 calories to your meal.

When you sit down, instruct the waiter not to bring any tortilla chips. If it's too hard to resist those crunchy, salty chips with the salsa—and who can, really?—don't even allow them on the table. A serving of 12 chips contains 139 calories, 7 grams of fat, and 19 grams of carbs. Instead, order an appetizer of ceviche (fish marinated in lime juice) or a shrimp cocktail.

Start your meal with a broth-based soup. Mexican appetizers like nachos and tostadas are so tempting, but really, all the oil and cheese make them not worth the splurge. The next time you're at your favorite Mexican spot, ask for the *sopa de lima*, a chicken and tomato soup that gets a little zip from added lime juice. Another option is tortilla soup, which has tomato, onion, and garlic puréed into chicken broth, and garnished with shredded chicken, lettuce, and avocado. It's customary for these soups to be garnished with tortilla chips—and sometimes even cheese—but you can ask the waiter to leave them out.

Fill up on chicken fajitas. The beef and chicken in fajitas are roasted and seasoned without fat to make them flavorful and light. Better yet, the fajitas come with a load of tasty bell peppers, onions, and other veggies. Just watch how many of the tortillas, which usually come on the side, you eat. Keep in mind that a 6-inch flour tortilla contains 16 grams of carbs, while a 13-inch tortilla contains 34 grams. If you're counting carbs and you have room in your plan for the tortillas, stick to one or two. If you have "filling" left after that, eat it on its own.

Order Mexican main-dish salads with caution—and hold the deep-fried taco shell. As is true of many Mexican specialties, main-dish salads are typically dressed up with high-fat cheese, avocado, and sour cream in addition to healthy ingredients like tomatoes, corn, and black beans. The worst health offender of all is the crispy, deep-fried taco shell that some salads are served in, which adds nearly 500 calories, 27 grams of fat, and 50 grams of carbohydrates to your meal. Your best course of action? Order the salad without the shell, and tell them to hold the cheese and sour cream.

Make your own main dish salad. Choose a lean dish on the menu, such as the fajitas or *pollo a la parilla* (grilled chicken), and ask for it to be served over greens. The restaurant may charge you a little extra but will probably oblige.

Top your burrito with salsa and a little guacamole, rather than sour cream and cheese. Fresh salsa delivers no fat and just 10 calories per tablespoon. On the other hand, sour cream is loaded with saturated fat—the kind that clogs your arteries and raises your cholesterol. And although guacamole is made with avocados, which are full of healthy monounsaturated fat, it's quite high in calories. If you keep the guacamole to a couple of table-spoons, you'll add only 4 grams of fat and 43 calories to your meal.

Skip the combo platters and order a la carte. They usually come with rice (which has 21 grams of carbohydrates in one serving) and refried beans (which contain 39 carbohydrates per cup and are sometimes made with artery-clogging lard). Good a la carte options include soft tacos with chicken, vegetables, or beef, or almost anything else that is baked or roast-ed (the word for "roasted" in Spanish is *asada)* and is not buried under a mound of cheese.

Plan a festive evening of dinner and dancing. Eating Mexican? Make a date to go salsa dancing after your meal. Not only will the prospect of postprandial activity inspire you not to gorge yourself, you'll burn off some of the calories you did eat. You'll certainly have a lot more fun than you would if you went home and watched TV! Not a danc-ing couple? Go hear a Mexican guitarist play, or hit a street fair with a Latin flair. Just keep the south-of-the-border theme going!

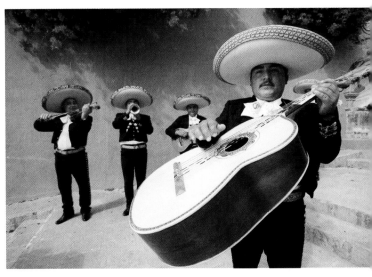

Order a naked chicken burrito. That is, a burrito without a tortilla. A giant tortilla can weigh in at more than 300 calories. Have the burrito without it—and without the cheese—and you'll likely get a meal (chicken, beans, salsa, and lettuce) that's reasonable in calories. Or order a regular burrito, cut it in half, and ask the waiter to wrap the rest.

indulging in Italian food

Making smart choices at an Italian restaurants boils down to this: Watch your servings of carbs from pizza and pasta, and steer clear of creamy, cheesy sauces and "stuffings." Fortunately, Italy's cuisine is healthy at heart. Big salads and antipasto are easy ways to squeeze in fresh vegetables, and at high-end Italian restaurants, fish is often on the menu.

Lean on Southern Italian cuisine. Southern Italy is famous for its olive oil and fresh seafood and vegetables, and its cuisine has much less butter, cream, and beef than that of its Northern neighbors. (That's not to say that they don't do pasta and pizza—they do; they're just vehicles for tomato-based sauces and veggies.)

Make protein the focal point of your entrée. When we think Italian food, we tend to focus on carb-dense offerings like pasta and pizza and forget all about their delectable meat dishes. For a real treat—and a real break for your blood sugar compared to the garlic bread and deep-dish pizza—try veal picatta, chicken or veal cacciatore, or the fish special of the day. Unlike carbohydrates, protein has almost no effect on blood sugar, and studies show it keeps you full longer than fat or carbs do.

Keep your pasta portions in check. Pasta isn't as bad for your blood sugar as we think it is—it's made from durum wheat, which is digested more slowly than, say, white bread and rice. But it's still high in carbohydrates (white pasta has about 15 grams of carbohydrate in just ⅓ cup), so you should limit your portions. A side serving of pasta should be just half a cup, and a main dish pasta should be no more than a cup (but is often twice that).

Order spaghetti topped with tomatoes, onions, garlic, and broccoli. Forget meat and cream-based sauces—make your next pasta dish work magic on your health. A study from India showed significant improvement

golden rule! **Top Pizza with at Least Two Vegetables**

Topping a slice of pizza with vegetables is not only an easy way to ramp up your veggie intake, it's also a smart, low-cal, low-fat alternative to meat toppings. So go for spinach, (a single ounce of which provides more than half of your daily requirements of vitamin A), bell peppers, onions, and sliced tomatoes. If you're making your own pizza, top it with raw chopped garlic; the sulfur compounds act as antioxidants, and the herb has a modest cholesterol-lowering effect.

in blood sugar levels of people who ate 2 ounces of onions a day. Other studies link garlic to increased insulin secretion and lower blood sugar, as well as increased levels of "good" cholesterol. Finally, the Centers for Disease Control and Prevention found that people with impaired glucose tolerance had lower levels of lycopene, a carotenoid found in tomatoes, than those without diabetes.

Tell your waiter that you don't want extra oil added to your pasta. It's not uncommon for restaurant kitchens to add a little olive oil to their noodles before they send them off to your table—it makes them taste better and keeps the pasta from sticking together. But at about 120 calories and 14 grams of fat per tablespoon, you'll be better off without it. How can you tell if they abided by your request? If the pasta looks shinier at the restaurant than it does when you make it at home, it's coated with oil.

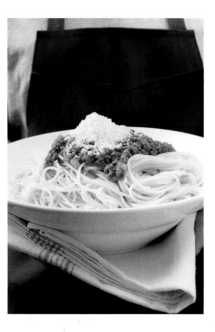

Choose red sauce over white. Making the right sauce selection is the single biggest health decision you'll make at an Italian restaurant, because the sauce you choose can either ensure a healthy meal or muck up the week's careful calorie and fat planning. Tomatoes—the backbone of marinara and puttanesca sauces—are a good source of vitamin C and lycopene. But if the sauce is white, as in fettuccine Alfredo, or even pink, as in penne a la vodka, it means that cream is playing a major role. A plate of spaghetti with plain tomato sauce contains just 440 calories and 5 grams of fat (1 gram of saturated fat). By contrast, the same size portion of fettuccine Alfredo packs 1,130 calories and 83 grams of fat, 51 of which are saturated.

Trade original-crust pizza for thin crust. Order a slice of thin-crust pizza instead of regular-crust pizza and you'll cut your carb grams in *half.* You'll also save 80 calories.

Watch for the "pizza effect." Because pizza contains a lot of carbs and also a lot of fat, which slows the rate at which the carbs are digested, it's notorious for causing a delayed rise in blood sugar. Every pizza is unique in the density of the crust, the sugar in the pizza sauce, and the amount of fat it contains, so the only way to know the effect of a particular pizza is to check your blood sugar two hours after a meal. You many discover that pizzas from different restaurants have different effects on blood sugar. The results also help you decide if you need to stop at one or two slices of pizza.

healthy eating on the go

Fast food is practically synonymous with "fat" food, and there's little doubt that our propensity for it has influenced the obesity epidemic. A study conducted at Boston Children's Hospital looked at more than 3,000 adults and found that those who said they visited fast-food restaurants more than twice a week gained about 10 pounds more weight than people who said they went less than once a week. They also had a twofold greater increase in insulin resistance. Fortunately, fast-food joints are finally stepping up and offering more healthy options. Here's how to navigate the fast-food jungle and come out unscathed.

Read the on-site nutrition information. Fast-food restaurants don't exactly advertise this fact because so many of their offerings are unhealthy, but most of them do have on-site poster-sized charts or brochures detailing their nutrition information. And seeing these numbers in black and white will show you how easy it is to trim calories and, say, order a regular hamburger at McDonald's (with 250 calories, 9 grams of fat, and 31 grams of carbohydrates) rather than a Quarter Pounder (which has 410 calories, 19 grams of fat, and 37 grams of carbohydrates). You can also do this research ahead of time at the company's Web site.

Keep nutrition guides to your favorite fast-food restaurants in your glove compartment. The next time you're pressed for time and have to order your lunch at a drive-through window, you'll have the calories, fat, and sodium figures at your fingertips.

Pass on the fried fish sandwich. These may sound healthier than burgers, but they're generally not. The Big Fish sandwich at Burger King contains 630 calories and 30 grams of fat (6 of them saturated). A Filet-O-Fish sandwich at McDonald's will give you 380 calories and 18 grams of total fat, 4 of them saturated.

Eat like a kid, not like a grownup. Ordering a child-size meal rather than an adult-sized combination meal is not just cheaper, it means eating half as many calories and grams of fat. For example, a McDonald's Happy Meal with a hamburger, small French fries, and 12-ounce soda contains 600 calories and 22 grams of fat. The adult version of the same meal— a Quarter Pounder without cheese, a large fries, and a 21-ounce soft drink—contains 1,190 calories and 49 grams of fat.

Order a grilled, not crispy, chicken sandwich. Chicken can certainly be a healthy fast-food option—that is, if you order the grilled version rather than the deep-fried cutlet. This easy decision saves you 10 grams of carbs (51 grams, compared to 61 in the fried chicken). The grilled chicken also has 80 fewer calories and 7 fewer grams of fat. Hold the mayo and save even more fat calories.

Wash down your meal with water or unsweetened iced tea instead of soda. Soda or sweetened drinks such as lemonade or iced tea are full of sugar and have no nutritional value. An 8-ounce glass of Coke carries 27 grams of carbs while 9 ounces of lemonade has 40 grams of carbs. If you must have a soda, make sure it's diet.

Give your bones a boost by ordering fat-free or 1 percent milk. Many fast-food restaurants now offer cartons of milk, and you know the calcium's good for your bones. But the milk may have other benefits as well, such as lowering your blood pressure and possibly even helping you lose weight. Also encourage family members who don't have diabetes to drink their milk. In a study of 10,000 women, those who consumed more calcium and vitamin D (which is in fortified milk) had a lower chance of developing metabolic syndrome, a cluster of symptoms that raise the chances of getting type 2 diabetes and heart disease.

Pass up the milkshakes. Some large fast-food milkshakes contain over 1,000 calories—more than the 640 calories in a small hamburger, small fries, and small Coke. To wash your burger down, order water, unsweetened tea, or low-fat milk.

Focus on garden-variety salads, not exotic ones. Surely you've seen television commercials for new, "healthy" fast-food salads: Some are Asian themed and come with crunchy noodles and Mandarin orange pieces, and others have crispy buffalo chicken pieces and cheese atop some greens. A quick glance at restaurants' nutrition data shows that these salads are sometimes more fatty and calorie-laden than the sandwiches and burgers! If nutritional information is not at hand, stick to salads that are full of veggies rather than cheese, croutons, "crispy" meats, and noodles. Also, choose a noncreamy dressing and use it sparingly.

golden rule! Remove Your "Healthy Halo"

When you feel righteous for ordering a turkey sandwich on wheat loaded with veggies and no mayo, you might feel like you have permission to get a bag of chips, a cookie, and soda, too. This "I made one healthy choice—I deserve it" feeling is what Vicki Saunders, RD, a nutrition educator at St. Helena Hospital in Napa Valley, California, calls a "healthy halo." Resist the urge to spend more calories than those you've saved, and instead give yourself a nonfood treat, like a long soak in the bathtub, for your "heavenly" behavior.

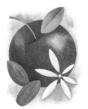

Simple switches can bring your sandwich back within healthy bounds.

making lean choices at the deli counter

Many people get their lunches from mom-and-pop sandwich shops because they perceive them as healthier alternatives to fast-food restaurants—and they can be, if you make the right choices. But the deli's breakfast sandwiches and foot-long, three-salami heroes can do more damage to your diet than a double cheeseburger. Here's how to eat lean and green at the corner deli.

Before you bite into a bagel, budget those carbs into your meal plan. A typical bakery bagel contains about 70 grams of carbohydrates—about five times as many carbs as a slice of whole-wheat bread (and more than four carb exchanges, for those who are counting). Research shows that the *amount* of carbohydrates, not the *kind* of carbohydrates, most influences the amount of glucose in the blood. Ingesting a whole bagel in one sitting may cause your blood sugar to spike; consider eating half of the bagel now, and half later in the day to spread your carb intake out.

Skip the salami and bologna. You'll blow your saturated fat and sodium allowance for much of the day. A single slice of beef bologna has 87 calories and 302 milligrams of sodium. Compare that to a slice of smoked turkey breast, with only 28 calories and 257 milligrams of sodium.

Ask for less meat and extra fixings. A serving size of deli meats is just two slices—a fraction of what delis usually give you. Ask them to cut the meat in half and bulk up your sandwich (and add extra flavor and crunch) with lettuce, tomatoes, hot peppers, onions, sprouts, and other veggies.

Hold the mayo, special sauce, and cheese. Even a lean turkey breast sandwich can be full of fat if you add on cheese and fattening condiments, says Molly Morgan, RD. "Some of the sub shops are famous for saying a sandwich has so many grams of fat, but that's without the cheese, mayo, and sauce," she explains. Simple switches can bring your sandwich back within healthy bounds: Substituting mustard for mayonnaise makes it 10 grams of fat lighter. Forgo vague-sounding "house" or "special" sauces, too, which are usually mayonnaise based.

Ask for a whole-wheat, rather than white, roll. Though the amount of carbs will be about the same as you'd get from a white roll, ordering the wheat will at least add 1 or 2 grams of fiber to your meal.

Or hold the roll altogether. Most sub shops will turn your favorite sub into a salad by tossing the meat and veggies onto a bed of lettuce rather than a roll. A six-inch Italian white sub roll can have 38 grams of carbs— a huge carb savings if you skip it. Have a piece of fruit instead.

put your beverages on a diet

Most of us would prefer to eat our calories than drink them. And studies have shown that even a high-calorie drink will never be as satisfying as something you bite into. Here's the skinny on how to keep your beverages from pushing an otherwise healthy meal into the caloric "red zone."

Beware of fancy water. These days, water isn't just water. Sometimes it comes in colors and has added vitamins, herbs, or caffeine. These designer waters are being positioned as a healthy alternative to regular bottled water or soft drinks. But are they worth the hefty price? Probably not. And many of these waters are not calorie free, as plain water is, so read the labels. One bottle may contain two servings, so don't forget to double the calorie count if you drink the whole thing.

Follow the 50/50 rule. If there's a fancy water or other drink you like that's a bit high in calories, go ahead and quaff it—after you dilute with an equal part regular water. Getting plenty of fluids into your body is important for everyone and especially for people with diabetes. It improves blood flow and helps the kidneys do their job of flushing toxins from the body. It could even lower your risk of diabetes-related kidney damage. So if you really dislike plain water and "flavoring" your water a bit with one of these drinks helps you drink more, by all means do it.

Is Coffee Okay?

Every other week, it seems, a new health report comes out about coffee. Studies have suggested that the beverage protects against certain cancers and Parkinson's disease, and it's one of the best sources of antioxidants in our diet (mainly because we drink so much of it). But there's more.

One of the compounds in coffee, called chlorogenic acid, has been shown in animal studies to lower blood sugar. Coffee's also rich in quinides, compounds that make the body more sensitive to insulin. These could be among the reasons why regular coffee drinkers seem to have a lower risk of developing diabetes. A survey of 80,000 women conducted by the Harvard School of Public Health showed that drinking two to three cups a day lowered the chance of developing type 2 diabetes by about a third.

So go ahead, join in a klatch at the local coffee shop—but stick to decaf, because caffeine can cause spikes in your blood sugar by raising so-called "stress" hormones that stimulate the release of stored glucose from the liver.

Grab unsweetened iced tea instead of soda. You'll not only save yourself the calories of regular soda, you'll also infuse your body with disease-fighting antioxidants.

Fade that coffee to black. Given the myriad flavors, fillers, and toppings you can add to coffee these days, black coffee may sound kind of plain—but it's practically calorie-free! A 12-ounce black coffee at Starbucks contains only 5 calories and 1 gram of carbohydrate, and a shot of espresso with a splash of milk has only 10 calories and 1 carb gram. The more you add to your java, the more those numbers go up: A shot of espresso sweetened with caramel and served with whipped cream has 110 calories and 9 grams of fat, 6 of which are saturated.

Order your java drinks "skinny." In coffee-shop lingo, "skinny" means, "made with skim milk," and folks who don't want to drink their calories are making the switch from "fat" to "skinny." Ordering a 16-ounce latte made with skim milk instead of whole milk will cut 110 calories out of the drink.

Treat fancy, specialty coffees as you would a dessert. The more flavors and toppings you add to a specialty coffee drink, the higher its calorie count climbs—so high, in some cases, that ordering an ice cream cone would be healthier. A sugar cone with half a cup of vanilla ice cream contains about 185 calories and 8 grams of fat (5 saturated). A 16-ounce cinnamon dolce frappuccino from Starbucks, which is a coffee with added sugar, whipped cream, and sprinkles, contains 420 calories, 16 grams of fat (10 saturated) and 61 grams of carbs. Even when you order the light version of the drink, you'll still be getting 41 grams of carbs and more than 300 calories. Always bear in mind that these drinks aren't refreshments—they're desserts—and should be consumed sparingly, on special occasions.

chapter eleven

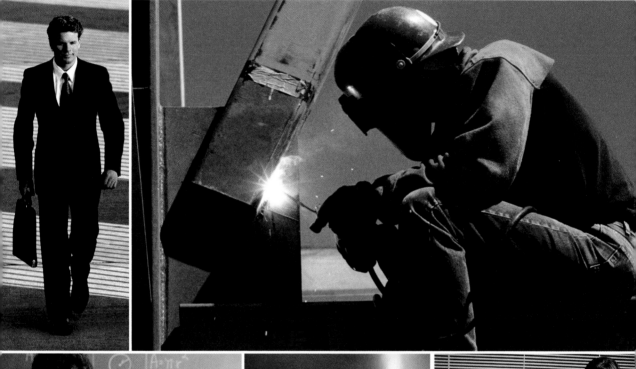

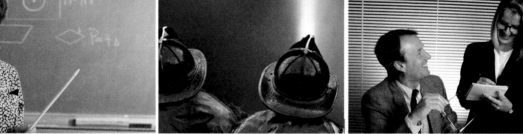

at work

When you head to work in the morning, you take your diabetes with you. Plan to treat it well by eating right, fitting in some exercise, and keeping stress under control while you're on the clock.

eating well at work

Depending on what you do for a living, you probably need certain tools to do your job: Maybe it's a hammer, computer, cell phone, or client database. Doubtless you'll also need a clear head—and that means steady blood sugar. Committing to eating wholesome meals and snacks at work may involve a little extra effort, but think of it as time devoted to satisfying your most important customer: your body!

Make your lunch while you make dinner. If your workplace cafeteria doesn't offer healthy options, you'll best meet your nutritional needs by bringing your own lunch. This isn't as much of a pain as it sounds—just make tomorrow's lunch tonight, while you're making dinner. You'll be in the kitchen anyway! One thing you can do is make an extra serving of your dinner and set it aside for the next day. If you don't want to eat the same thing two days in a row, do something new with the main dinner ingredient. For example, slice some of the roasted chicken you just made and tuck it into a whole-wheat pita with some onion and apple slices, or toss it in with some whole-wheat pasta and broccoli.

While you're in the kitchen, pack a few snacks. Why resort to vending-machine junk when you can bring your own, more gourmet bites? Throw a few items such as low-fat mozzarella cheese sticks, hummus, sliced apples, mandarin oranges, and fruit and yogurt into plastic containers, stow them in your lunch sack, and keep the sack in the refrigerator. The whole exercise takes less than five minutes and saves you the hassle of doing it the next morning.

Carry a cool lunch sack. If you don't have a refrigerator at your worksite, that doesn't mean you can't bring a perishable lunch to work. With an insulated lunch bag, you can bring chilled meals and snacks to work that will keep until you eat them. Check out a well-stocked kitchen or gift store; men can find sacks that are just as masculine as the old-fashioned metal

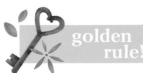

golden rule! ## Eat as Healthfully at Work as You Would at Home

The calories and fat you eat outside your home count just as much as those you consume under your own roof—so why is it that you watch your Ps and Qs when you cook your own meals and forget them when you're at work? Get into the habit of bringing both a homemade lunch *and* a take-charge attitude to work with you. Tell yourself that you're going to feel great 'round the clock, not just when you're off the clock.

whip it together! Brown Bag Chili

Why settle for a cold sandwich when you can have a hot lunch from home? This one's full of protein to keep you full all day.

Mince 3 **scallions** and 2 **garlic** cloves. In a large saucepot sauté them in 2 teaspoons of **canola oil** for 3 minutes. Add 1 tablespoon **chili powder** and 1 teaspoon ground **cumin**. Add 1 pound lean **ground turkey or chicken**. Brown for 5 minutes over medium heat. Add 1 can (15 ounces) drained and rinsed **kidney beans** and 1 can (14½ ounces) no-salt-added **stewed tomatoes**. Simmer for 5 minutes. Spoon into a thermos and refrigerate. Reheat prior to serving.

lunchboxes, and women can buy insulated sacks that look just like cute handbags or tote bags.

Grill a dietitian for gourmet lunch suggestions. If eating the same snacks and lunches day in and day out is testing your fortitude, schedule a visit with a registered dietitian. These nutritional professionals have tons of creative ideas about healthy, time-saving snacks and meals you can bring to work, no matter what your schedule or workplace setup is. They'll even take into account the foods you like most.

Organize a weekly "soup club" with your coworkers. Everyone likes soup, and most people have a favorite soup recipe at home. Once a week, have everyone who signs up for the club bring enough soup for all. Just be sure to set these ground rules: no cream, no coconut milk, and not too much salt. The cook should also bring in enough copies of the recipe for everyone.

"Lunchpool" with three health-conscious colleagues. "Lunchpooling" is like carpooling, but for meal preparation: Band together with a few friends who are tired of the hassle of bringing their lunch every day, and assign each person a day of the week. On their assigned days, "lunchpool" club members will prepare a healthy meal that will feed all four people in the club. It's less cooking for everyone involved and a fun opportunity to try some new dishes you might want to rotate into your own menu.

Highlight healthy options on your favorite takeout menus. It happens all the time—someone comes around with a takeout menu and invites you to order. And of course the menu is full of choices that would blow your entire fat, calories, and salt allotment for the rest of the day. No problem— that's precisely why you've done your homework and identified two or three dishes that won't sabotage your eating plan. Ask for one of those dishes and you won't even have to look temptation in the face.

resisting tempting treats on the job

In a 2006 survey conducted by Careerbuilder.com, nearly half of all workers reported that they had gained weight since starting their present jobs. And it's easy to see why: We all give in to vending machines, bowls of candy on coworkers' desks, and office birthday cake. And if you're sitting behind a desk all day, the pounds seem to sneak up on you even faster. Because excess weight is a problem for so many people with diabetes, resisting the small temptations at work will go a long way toward helping you manage your condition.

Spend your downtime in a snack-free break area. The snacks that you'll likely find in the break room can make it one of the most dangerous areas at your workplace. Scout out another quiet spot where you can retreat during your downtime. This can be a shady area under some trees behind the building, a file room with a chair, or an unused office with a pleasant view. When your usual break room is laden with doughnuts and cookies that your coworkers have brought in, sneak away to your special spot.

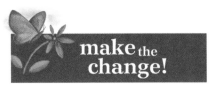

The habit: Choosing pretzels instead of corn chips from the vending machine.

The result: Losing about 5 pounds a year.

The proof: Although they may seem like the same kind of snack—they're both tasty and crunchy—pretzels are a much better vending choice than flavored tortilla chips. A typical 1.5-ounce bag of pretzels from a vending machine contains about 180 calories and 1.5 grams of fat, but a 1.75-ounce bag of nacho-cheese corn chips has 250 calories and 13 grams of fat. If you picked the pretzels instead of the chips every workday, after a year you'd save about 18,500 calories. That's the equivalent of 5 pounds of body weight! You'd save yourself a considerable amount of artery-clogging saturated fat, too.

Sip cool water throughout the day. Bring two 32-ounce bottles of water to work each morning, and make it a goal to drink them before you go home. This is important for a few reasons: Being dehydrated can cause your blood sugar to rise. Also, water is filling so you'll feel less hungry during the day. Research shows that drinking at least 50 ounces of cold water can burn 50 extra calories each day, because you have to expend energy to bring the water up to body temperature. Do this for a year and you'll lose about 5 pounds, not counting the calories you're *not* ingesting by drinking soda.

Give your water a zing of fruit flavor. At the beginning of the workweek, bring several sliced limes or lemons in a resealable plastic bag and store them in the refrigerator at work. When you refill your water bottle, squeeze some juice into the bottle, then toss the slice in. For variety, try dropping slices of cucumber, strawberries, or sprigs of mint into your water. It's like having a spa treat at your desk!

Stock your desk or locker with a variety of teas. Sipping hot tea is an easy way to drink a lot of water and feel full while you work. Green or black teas are also two of the most potent sources of antioxidants in nature, and sipping them regularly has been shown to decrease the risk of heart disease and stroke, to which people with diabetes are more susceptible. For the sake of your blood pressure, choose decaffeinated tea (you'll still get the antioxidants). Store the tea bags inside an airtight container, in a cool, dry place (a desk drawer is ideal).

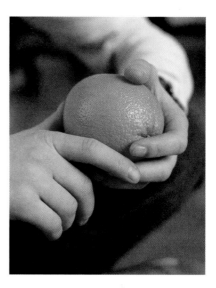

Do some "home cooking" from your desk. If there's no microwave in the break room (and if it's okay with your supervisor), keep an electric hot pot in your workspace. You can use it to heat water for tea, which will help you stay hydrated throughout the day. Because you can also reheat food in it (like a can of low-sodium soup, or last night's stew), a hot pot can also make eating healthy lunches easier.

Hide your own stash of healthy snacks. You'll have no excuse to hit the vending machine when a snack craving strikes! Nonperishable nibbles like small boxes of high-fiber cereal, packets of instant oatmeal, low-fat crackers, small cans of fruit packed in their own juice, and trail mix are good choices to keep in your drawer. If you have a refrigerator at work, keep some low-fat cheese sticks and low-fat yogurt in there.

Keep sugarless mints and gum in your drawer, and chew on one when temptation hits. If you're due at a meeting in 10 minutes and you know there will be doughnuts or cookies on the table, pop a couple of breath mints or a piece of chewing gum into your mouth before you head over. The mint's strong flavor ruins the taste of anything that you eat, especially sugary baked goods. It's a bonus that your breath smells sweet while you're talking business!

Focus on your food when you're eating. You get more work done when you focus on your tasks; similarly, you'll get more flavor and enjoyment out of your snacks and meals if you turn all of your attention to the food in front of you. Don't work or browse the Internet as you eat. Sit outside under a tree, or turn off your computer monitor and look out the window while you eat—then you're not only enjoying your food, you're also de-stressing a bit.

Indulge in a nonedible distraction. When your coworkers are celebrating someone's birthday with a gigantic cake, the cut-up veggies that you're keeping in the office fridge aren't going to keep you from joining in the feeding frenzy. But engaging in more meaningful distractions—ones that

whip it together! Tote-Along Bagel Chips

When the afternoon munchies strike, reach for these homemade bagel chips, which are much lower in calories and fat than store-bought ones.

Preheat the oven to 425°F. Slice one **whole-wheat bagel** horizontally into 4 slices. Cut each of the slices into 6 pieces. Spread the bagel pieces onto a large baking sheet and spray them with butter or olive oil cooking spray. In a small bowl combine 2 tablespoons grated **Parmesan cheese**, 1 tablespoon dried **basil**, 2 teaspoons dried **oregano**, 2 teaspoons **garlic powder**, 1 teaspoon **onion powder**, and **salt** and **pepper** to taste. Sprinkle the chips with the herb mixture. Bake for about 5 to 6 minutes until lightly toasted. Pack into a zip-close bag.

have nothing to do with food—might keep you from overindulging. If your workplace allows it, spend five minutes surfing the Internet to read about a new movie you want to see, or phone a friend or your spouse for a quick hello. While your coworkers are chowing down, you'll be reaffirming your commitment to making healthy lifestyle choices.

Prepare a polite response to pushy coworkers. Every day, or so it seems, well-meaning coworkers proffer homemade muffins or candies they picked up on vacation, and sometimes it's just easier to eat up rather than hurt your friend's feelings. Having a kind "no" prepared in advance can keep those sugary treats from sending your blood sugar levels soaring: Try, "No thanks, I've already been snacking at my desk," or, "I appreciate the offer, but I have a delicious dinner planned for tonight, so I'm saving room for that."

If you just can't curb that snack attack, at least petition snack vendors for healthier treats. Your office's vending machine doesn't have to be a nutritional wasteland! Ask the company that stocks the machine to provide some healthy options. Be specific about what you want: Ask for particular brands of chips and other snacks that you know are low-calorie, such as pretzels and baked, rather than fried, tortilla chips (and maybe ask that snacks that contain trans fat be banished). If you think management would be amenable, petition higher-ups for a refrigerated vending machine stocked with options like fresh fruit and yogurt.

Brush and floss your teeth after meals and snacks. It's another good reason to get up from your desk, and you'll be doing your mouth a favor, since people with diabetes are at higher risk of gum disease. Brushing up will also make you less tempted to eat again later in the day.

putting your company's resources to work for you

It's in your company's best interest to encourage you to exercise, lose weight, and get regular medical checkups. A healthy employee is happier, more productive, more energetic, and takes fewer sick days. As a result, businesses are offering more and more programs to help their workers track and improve their health. Take full advantage.

Take advantage of corporate health screenings. Some businesses host health screenings regularly and invite nurses and other health professionals to come to the office and check employees' blood pressure and cholesterol, administer flu shots, perform skin-cancer screenings, and more. Find out when these screenings will take place in your office, and be sure to sign up. Everyone with diabetes should get a flu shot every year, and keeping tabs on your blood pressure and cholesterol are especially important if you have diabetes because of the increased risk of heart attack and stroke that comes with the disease.

Learn whether your company offers incentives to exercise. Some companies offer reduced fees at the local gym or reimbursement for sports lessons. It doesn't hurt to ask, and if your company doesn't offer these incentives yet, maybe you'll inspire them to start.

Suggest ways to make your worksite healthier. Your boss knows that happy, healthy employees are more productive employees. Why wouldn't he be interested in your suggestions for improving the workplace, particularly if they don't cost much? If the cafeteria offers too many fried foods and not enough vegetables, suggest specific improvements. Or come up with ways that the company could make healthy living in the workplace more prevalent—perhaps by organizing walking groups or hosting a guest speaker during lunch hour. Your career may benefit, too, because you'll be seen as a team player with creative problem-solving skills.

Start a good-natured weight-loss competition. What's the surest way to cut down on the amount of junk food that's brought into the office? Engage in a little competition with your coworkers over who can lose the most weight—and put a wager on it, if it's not against office policy. You might even organize colleagues into teams, or by department: Pit the crew in the mailroom against the staffers in accounting, for example. Hold weekly check-in meetings during which you and your teammates offer each other encouragement and weight-loss strategies. You'll be less likely to indulge in doughnuts or coffee cake at your next morning meeting if you know that your team is counting on you to make healthy choices.

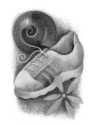

Take advantage if your company offers reimbursement for gym member fees.

stay active while on the clock

These days, it's all too common to sit at a desk for the better part of eight hours a day—something the human body just wasn't designed to do. Even if you're getting plenty of exercise in the evenings and on weekends, moving around at work is essential: It can help prevent stiff and sore joints, give your eyes a break from the computer monitor, and give you enough adrenaline to stay focused and energized throughout the day.

Pedal to work. Your daily trip to the office presents a great opportunity to burn calories while you escape the stressful car commute. If you don't live far from work, pick one day a week or month and pedal to work. If you bicycle at an average speed of 12 miles an hour—a brisk pace, but reasonable for many people—you'll burn about 410 calories an hour. Before you begin riding to work, ask your city parks or transportation department for a map of safe bike routes in your city. Check traffic and street conditions before you leave the house, wear a helmet, and find a secure place at work to lock your bike.

Keep a pair of athletic shoes and socks under your desk or in your locker. When an opportunity to get even a little extra exercise arises during the day—if your boss sends you on an errand, or you have to lend a hand in the company warehouse—you'll be ready to lace up your shoes and get moving. If you're worried about theft, keep an older pair of shoes at work, as long as they are comfortable and have some life left in them.

Bowl with your accounting buddies. Many workplaces use sports as team-building experiences and sponsor company softball, volleyball, bowling, or golf teams. These activities are great ways to burn calories; they also give you a chance to network with coworkers and supervisors during games and practices. Ask around at your office to learn what sorts of team sports your coworkers play. Be sure to find out how competitively the team plays, and decide if your fitness level and intensity are a good match for the team. Some teams just hit the field to have a good time, but some company teams take the game very seriously and expect everyone to play to win.

Deliver important messages in person. Rather than sending an impersonal e-mail or making a phone call,

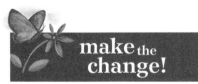

make the change!

The habit: Wearing comfortable, easy-to-move-in clothes.

The result: Keeping your weight under control.

The proof: Research has found that employees take 491 more steps during the workday when they're wearing casual clothing than when they're wearing business attire. If your company doesn't permit you to wear casual clothing every day, wear clothes that are as comfortable as your company's dress code will allow. Look for garments that feel cool while you're moving around and don't restrict your movements, and wear comfortable shoes that encourage walking. On casual Fridays and other dress-down days, be sure you do extra physical activity to take advantage of the comfortable clothes. By taking just 491 extra steps each day, you can burn nearly 2 pounds a year!

Easy Moves to Do at Your Desk

Simple exercises to stretch and strengthen your muscles at your desk not only burn calories, they help you feel refreshed and limber throughout the day, which will give you enough energy to exercise after work. Each morning and afternoon, do at least one of these exercises:

• **Leg lifts.** Keeping one foot on the ground, lift the other leg off the ground a few inches. Raise and lower the leg 10 to 20 times, then switch legs and repeat on the other side.

• **Desk pulls.** If you have a chair with rollers, pull your chair close to your desk, then slowly push yourself out to arm's length. Grip the desk tightly and pull yourself slowly back to the desk until your chest is touching it. Repeat 10 to 15 times.

• **Shoulder shrugs.** Many of us carry lots of tension in our shoulders due to stress. This exercise can help relieve that tension. Slowly lift your shoulders toward your ears, hold for a few seconds, and slowly lower them. Repeat 10 times.

get up at least once an hour and talk over work issues (or bring important papers along) in person. When your message is especially sensitive or personal, or when body language really matters, the in-person strategy is most important. Making these trips may only get you on your feet for five minutes, but those minutes add up over the course of a week.

If you have an office with a door, close it and jog in place for five minutes. For more of a challenge, jog in place and try to kick your butt as you do it, alternating legs (do this for 15 seconds, then rest for 30 seconds). Jumping jacks work well, too. You'll burn some calories and, chances are, you'll be much more energized when you return to your work.

On your way home, work out in the car. Yes, it's possible. First, tense and relax your leg muscles for about 10 seconds. Next, tighten and relax your buttocks for the same amount of time. Do the same with your abdominal and chest muscles. Finally, tense your arms against the resistance of the steering wheel. Now that most people drive at least a half hour to get to work, you'll have plenty of time to do these isometric exercises without taking up any time in your day, and you'll slowly get fitter.

managing work-related stress

They don't call it "work" for nothing. Every day there are different challenges to cope with, from meeting tight deadlines to dealing with difficult people. But when you have diabetes, hassles at work can be detrimental to your health. Stress can make your blood sugar go up or down and contributes to higher blood pressure, which raises the risk of heart disease and stroke. It can also weaken your resolve to eat healthy and exercise. Use these tips to ensure that your time at work is peaceful, productive, and conducive to living well with diabetes.

Schedule difficult tasks when you're likely to feel your best. Most of us know the time of day when we're most productive—some of us come alive at 4 p.m., while others are at their best in the earliest hours of the day. Whenever possible, schedule your most important work tasks during your most productive, alert times. These are the times to be making sales calls, coming up with creative ideas for a marketing campaign, or pitching new ideas to your boss. When you're grumpy or in a nonproductive slump, answer low-priority e-mails and do your filing or record-keeping.

Tackle procrastination by breaking big projects into smaller steps. When you're facing a huge project and don't know where to begin, make a to-do list of small milestones that need to be met, and give yourself a deadline for completing each one. Each day, pick out a task that you'll complete to make sure you accomplish *something* toward your goal.

Take a few minutes to chat. Successful work relationships often depend on appreciating the other person, and that's much easier to do if you get to know them a bit on a personal level. So build a few minutes into your morning in which you spend a little social time with colleagues. Keep it short, but don't miss this opportunity to share a laugh or story.

Cultivate one or two work friends. You know it instinctively, and science has proven it: Friends make life (including work life) less stressful. Having social support at work is associated with lower blood pressure during

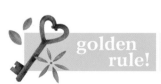

golden rule! Walk Every Day during Your Lunch Hour

Just 10 minutes of brisk walking could lower your blood sugar and will burn about 50 calories. Instead of chatting with coworkers after you're done eating, slip on your workout shoes and invite them to join you in a walk around the building. If the weather's bad, walk up and down the office stairs. It'll also do wonders for your soaring stress levels!

the workday and also with smaller increases in blood pressure during those times when work problems boil to a head.

Try a little aromatherapy at your desk. Studies have shown that pleasing, natural smells can relieve stress, especially when the scents are associated with positive memories. Scents that are best known for their stress-reducing qualities include lavender, ylang ylang, geranium, lemon, and roman chamomile. Fill a dish on your desk with potpourri, bring in a scented candle (but don't light it), or buy a fresh bouquet of flowers and place them in a vase on your desk every Monday.

Bring in several green plants. Choose ones that will survive well indoors. Studies find that plants significantly lower workplace stress and enhance productivity. Just the act of watering them can provide a brief, quiet moment of calm during your day.

Get a daily dose of inspiration from your computer. If your employer allows you to look at personal e-mail at work, sign up for a free service that will regularly send you motivational messages to help you with weight loss, exercise, or healthy eating. (Sign up through a personal e-mail account that you can access from your work computer, rather than using your work account.) Spending just a few moments reading these messages during your lunch hour or afternoon break can give you an encouraging boost that lasts the rest of the day.

Give yourself a pat on the back. When you've completed a goal, tell yourself what a good job you've done—and mean it. Praise is often in short supply on the job, so when you have a chance to praise yourself, take it. You'll get a burst of energy and confidence that will help you weather whatever storms the day has in store.

Pat others on the back, too (figuratively speaking). Don't hesitate to give praise and recognition, or even a simple compliment, to colleagues when appropriate. Making someone else feel good makes you feel good, too. And someday they may return the favor.

make the change!

The habit: Taking a walk instead of eating a candy bar.

The result: More energy and less tension.

The proof: In a study by researchers at California State University in Long Beach, participants either ate a candy bar or walked briskly for 10 minutes. The candy bar eaters felt tenser in the next hour, while the walkers experienced higher energy levels *and* reduced stress.

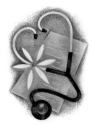

Teach a coworker symptoms of trouble and how to help in an emergency.

sharing your diabetes with your colleagues

Many workers with diabetes face a tough decision: Do they tell their bosses and coworkers about their medical condition or keep quiet about it? Regardless of which path you take, it's wise to give some thought to how you'll deal with delicate situations that arise on the job concerning your diabetes.

Train a trusted ally to help you in an emergency. If you're at risk of hypoglycemia, which may develop if you use insulin or glucose-lowering drugs, someone at your workplace needs to know how to help you should the situation arise. Enlist the aid of a colleague who's discreet, works nearby, and is able to solve problems calmly. Discuss the noticeable symptoms you may have, such as anxiety, irritability, or uncoordinated movements. Show your "helper" where you store your rescue foods to raise your blood sugar, and make sure you always keep them there. If your doctor has prescribed glucagon for emergencies, teach your helper how to inject it should you pass out, and keep the medication where your coworker can find it quickly.

Prepare a polite reply for coworkers who dispense medical advice. If you tell your colleagues that you have diabetes, be prepared to be on the receiving end of unsolicited advice from these armchair physicians. To discourage the receptionist's review of the miracle diabetes cure she saw on late-night TV, have a polite response at the ready. Try, "Thanks for sharing. My doctor and my dietitian keep me pretty well-informed on all the steps I should take." Or, "Thanks for your concern, but my diabetes is already under good control."

Before accepting a new job offer, imagine coping with your condition in the new setting. If you have nerve damage in your feet, a job that requires you to stand all day may not be the most comfortable choice. Because having a bout of low blood sugar may present safety issues, think hard about whether you want to be a heavy equipment operator. Make sure that you fully understand the schedule and the job requirements before you make any career-changing decisions. Be sure to investigate whether your diabetes qualifies as a "precondition," which might affect the health care coverage you receive through your new employer.

It's your choice whether or not to tell your employer you have diabetes. In general, your supervisors can only ask you about any medical issues if they believe you have a condition that's causing changes in your job performance, or if a medical condition may pose a safety risk in the workplace.

testing and injecting at work

File this paper, ring up a customer, finish this report. You have plenty of important tasks to handle during the course of a workday, but keeping your blood sugar steady should be a high priority, too. Checking your glucose and giving yourself injections during the day can fit easily into your schedule with just a little planning.

Be discreet when doing blood sugar checks and injections. You probably don't think much about checking your blood glucose or even giving yourself insulin—these are just routine activities, like tying your shoes. But your coworkers may be uncomfortable at seeing you draw the tiniest drop of blood or injecting yourself with a syringe. You shouldn't be ashamed about doing what you have to do to keep yourself healthy, but you should be mindful of actions that could make your colleagues uncomfortable.

Keep your glucose checking on schedule by setting an alarm. When you're already working on deadline and taking care of workplace emergencies that pop up, you may neglect checking your glucose regularly. If your glucose monitor has an alarm that beeps on a particular schedule when it's time for you to use it, make sure the alarm is set and the monitor is located where you can hear it. If your monitor doesn't have an alarm—or you don't want your coworkers to know about it—use a popup reminder on your computer's calendar, or wear a watch with an alarm that beeps.

Keep testing, eating, and medicine schedules for every shift you work. If your shifts vary between days and nights, you already know how hard it is to adjust your sleep schedule. But you'll also have to adjust the routine that you keep to monitor your blood sugar. In a notebook, write your schedule of checking your blood sugar, meal times, and medication usage when you're working a day shift. On another page, write a schedule

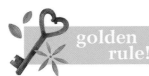

golden rule!   Keep a Stash of "Rescue" Foods Ready

If you're at risk for developing dangerously low blood sugar, keep foods that can raise your blood sugar quickly nearby in an easily accessed place so you (or someone else) can find them in an emergency. These might include hard candy or a bottle of juice. Glucose tablets are another option.

for the night shift. If you need help planning your schedules, talk to your doctor.

Carry your sharps home in a protective container. Use a portable sharps container at work to hold your used lancets, syringes, and insulin-pen needles. Tossing these into a trash can poses a safety hazard to your fellow employees, and it probably discloses more information about your health condition than your coworkers need to know. Containers specially designed for sharps are inexpensive and will fit into your purse or briefcase. Keep the container in your desk or other private area, and take them home to dispose of them properly.

If you use insulin, consider an insulin pen. Disposable (pre-filled) pens may be more convenient for you than syringes if you're injecting at work or on the go. (Note that not all insulin pens are disposable; the ones that aren't require you to replace the insulin cartridge once it's empty.) Pre-filled pens are small and discreet, and you can keep the pen you're currently using at room temperature. Once you've used up the insulin in the pen, you throw the pen away. You will need to screw on a new pen needle every time you inject. Ask your doctor if the type of insulin you need comes in a pre-filled pen.

If you need accommodations to cope with your diabetes on the job, ask. Your employer should be willing to make adjustments so you can get your job done, as long as they're not too difficult or expensive to implement. Reasonable requests might include a place to store food or inject insulin or a little flexibility to allow you to take a short break during the day if you come in early or stay late.

chapter twelve

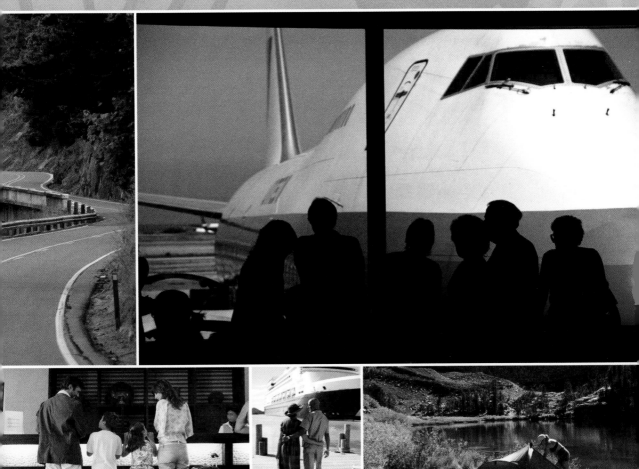

on the road

We call traveling "getting away from it all," but that doesn't mean you should take a break from healthy-living habits. Here's how to enjoy your trip, whether it's long or short, *and* stay on course.

in the driver's seat

There's nothing like a road trip to get you out of town in a hurry—just load up the car and go. But you'll want to shield yourself from some of the hazards inherent in road travel, from boredom to gas-station junk food to driving difficulties. Keep these tips in mind to arrive at your destination safe, alert, and refreshed.

Stash nourishment in your cup holders. Before you leave the house for that day trip to the zoo, fill a plastic drinking cup with sliced carrots and other veggies, or whole-wheat pita chips. Put some low-fat dip or hummus in another cup. Set these in the cup holders next to your seat—it's that easy to enjoy a diabetes-friendly snack while you're on the road.

For longer trips, buy a 9-quart cooler and pack it with healthy snacks. Junk food is doubly tempting when you're traveling by car: You're confined in a small space without much to do, and every time you stop for gas you keep thinking about how good a bag of salty chips and a cold soda would be. Having the right cooler—and stocking it well—can save you thousands of calories and hundreds of fat grams, not to mention money. These are the perfect size to fit behind the passenger seat of your car. Fill it with bottled water, precut carrots, red pepper slices, fruit, low-fat cheese sticks, and containers of low-fat dip, yogurt, or hummus. Top these items with a thick layer of ice. Put whole-wheat crackers sealed in zip-close bags on top.

Arm yourself with sandwiches. Your cooler can save you from more than the convenience store—it can also protect you from those ubiquitous fast-food joints and the crowds they're jammed with. Before you go, tuck turkey and sun-dried tomatoes with a dollop of spicy mustard into pita-bread pockets, or make a wrap sandwich with grilled chicken breast, spinach leaves, and red onion topped with zesty salsa and low-fat sour cream in a whole-wheat flour tortilla.

whip it together! Garlic-and-Onion Roasted Edamame

Instead of chips, try these crunchy, protein-rich snacks. Most supermarkets stock edamame, or green soybeans, in the frozen-foods section.

Toss 12 ounces shelled **edamame** with 2 teaspoons **olive oil,** ½ teaspoon each **garlic** and **onion powder,** ½ teaspoon **dried basil,** ¼ teaspoon **salt,** and ⅛ teaspoon **black pepper.** Roast on a baking sheet at 400°F for 10 minutes or until edamame looks dry and lightly browned. Store in zip-close bags.

golden rule!   Don't Leave Your Diabetes at Home

When it comes to managing your diabetes, your body doesn't care if you're on vacation or at home. The same standards for checking your blood sugar, eating healthy meals at regular intervals, and getting at least 30 minutes of physical activity every day still apply. Follow them and you'll feel better because your blood sugar will stay under control—and your trip will be less likely to be marred by a diabetes-related incident.

Bring along an audiobook. Reading is a sure way to make long drives pass quickly, but many bookworms in the passenger seat get motion sickness, and of course reading isn't an option for the driver. Before you leave for your trip, hit your bookstore or local library and buy or rent some audiobooks, or go online to sites such as itunes.com or audible.com. You'll find plenty of thrillers, romances, biographies, and humorous books to enrich your drive. If you're Web-savvy, you can download books to your digital audio player. These handy devices can hold a shelf's worth of books, and you can connect the player to your car's stereo.

Keep low blood sugar from becoming a highway hazard. Having low blood sugar while you're driving can endanger you and other motorists. If you ever feel the symptoms (such as dizziness, sweating, shakiness, and confusion) while you're behind the wheel, pull over as soon as you safely can. Check your blood sugar, and if it's low, drink a regular soda or juice, or eat some hard candy or glucose tablets. Wait 15 minutes and check your blood sugar again. You should resume driving only when your blood sugar level is within the normal range.

Seek medical professionals' advice on driving safely. Diabetes can cause several health issues that affect your driving ability, namely, blurry vision and nerve problems in your feet that can make it difficult to work the gas and brake pedals. Be sure to see your eye doctor at least once a year, and have your primary care physician check your feet regularly. If you think that vision problems or foot numbness are already interfering with your ability to drive, an occupational therapist or a driver rehabilitation specialist may help you learn how to compensate for these issues. Talk to your doctor or visit the Association for Driver Rehabilitation Specialists (www.driver-ed.org) to find the names of professionals in your area who can provide this instruction.

traveling with medicine and supplies

When it comes to your diabetes medications and injection supplies, "traveling light" can lead to heavy regret. If you rely on these items to keep your diabetes under control while you're at home, you're also going to need them while you're on the road.

Pack at least three days' extra supply of medication. That way you'll be covered in the event of car trouble, airport delays, or an unexpectedly fabulous time that makes you want to stay a day or two longer. (If you're running out of room in your satchel, leave an extra outfit at home—not your insulin.) If you're embarking on a long trip and want to bring more than a few days' supply of extra meds, ask your doctor if he can prescribe more than the typical one-month supply so you'll have enough extra to bring, and find out if your insurance company will cover it.

Bring extra batteries. Put fresh batteries into your glucose meter and, if you use one, your insulin pump. Estimate how many batteries these gadgets will need over the course of your trip, and bring twice that number. Tape the batteries into a little bundle, put them in a zip-close bag, and pack them in your shaving kit or cosmetics bag where they'll be easy to find.

Carry insurance against hypoglycemia. If your doctor has recommended that you keep glucagon handy to treat emergency episodes of low blood

A Primer for Your Travel Partner

Managing diabetes can be a two-person job when you're away from home. Here are a few pointers that will help your travel buddy help you stay healthy while traveling.

• **Show your companion where you keep your diabetes medications.** They can remind you where you've stowed them and can fetch them for you if you're unable to do so.

• **Teach your "assistant" the signs of hypoglycemia,** which can occur almost without warning if you get too much physical activity, don't eat enough, or take too much insulin or diabetes medication. These symp-toms include confusion, dizziness, sweating, and shaking. Instruct your companion to quickly bring you a regular soda, hard candy, or a small bottle of fruit juice to help you get your blood sugar back up quickly.

• **Give your pal permission to cajole you into making healthy choices** during your trip. These might include encouraging you to walk on the beach instead of napping on your beach towel, sharing a dessert rather than eating a whole one, and reminding you to check your blood pressure sooner rather than later.

sugar, be sure to bring it on your trip. Just as important, make sure your traveling companion knows how to administer it. If you are coherent enough to give yourself a shot of glucagon, you can probably treat the hypoglycemia by eating or drinking carbohydrates.

On long flights, be prepared to modify your insulin use. Consult a map that's marked with time zones and count the number of zones you'll be crossing to get to your destination. If you're heading west, your day will be longer and you may need more insulin injections. If you're flying east, your day will be shorter and you may need fewer. If you have any confusion on how to adapt your injection schedule during your flight, discuss the time zone difference with your doctor at your pre-trip visit.

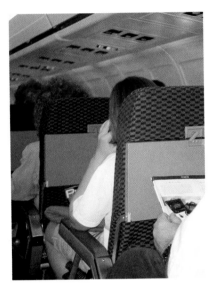

Carry your medication or equipment in its original packaging. Bring the original manufacturer's labels with your insulin, syringes and pens, testing equipment, and insulin pump and pump supplies. You may have trouble getting your medicine past the airport security if you don't have a properly labeled insulin bottle or the box your supplies came in. If carrying these items in their original boxes takes up too much space in your bag, pack the items outside of their boxes, flatten the boxes, and pack them flat in your carryon baggage. If a security checker is curious about your supplies, this info will help identify them.

Speak up before you get patted down. Tell the screeners at the airport security gate that you're carrying diabetes supplies, and carry the accompanying label information in hand along with your boarding pass; being ready will get you through the checkpoint without incident. If you use an insulin pump, ask that they visually inspect it.

Protect yourself and others from pokes. Tuck a one-quart "sharps" container designed for traveling into a carry-on bag or the glove box of your car so you can stash your used needles and lancets until you get home and can dispose of them safely. Small containers with puncture-proof walls and tightly fitting lids are available from drugstores.

Guard your insulin from temperature extremes. They can affect how well the insulin works. If you're walking or biking on a hot day, for example, put your insulin vial in an insulated tote bag to keep it cool. When traveling in the car, keep your insulin off the dashboard and out of the glove box. If you're cross-country skiing or hiking in the cold, keep the insulin in a pocket next to your body.

smart things to bring

Smart traveling is all about keeping yourself as comfortable and safe as possible while you enjoy your trip. These items can save you from blisters and foot injuries, help you out in an emergency, and more.

Get a note from your doc. Before your trip, visit your doctor and ask for a signed note on his letterhead that confirms your diagnosis, the generic and trade names for the medications you're taking, and your need for lancets, syringes, an insulin pump, or any other supplies you use. These documents will help you contact your physician in a pinch and may help out in case of an emergency or a problem with your medication.

Ask for an extra prescription. It's smart to get extra insulin or other medications you use in case you run out while you're on the road.

Pack two pairs of comfortable shoes. This way you can air one pair out while you tool around town in the other. Also bring a pair of brown or black, closed-toe flats for dinners and other more formal occasions. All the shoes you bring should be broken in before your trip, so leave your new ones at home.

Bring aqua shoes for the beach. These stretchy-soled booties will protect your feet from hot sand, rough sidewalks around the pool, and sharp pebbles underfoot.

Throw in an insulated tote. These bags are lined with a special material that keeps your food cool; you can find them near the insulated coolers in your local discount store. Before you set out for the day, stop by a deli and put a few cold bottles of water in the bag—they'll help keep everything else in the bag cool. Then add snacks like yogurt cups, sliced apples, and low-fat mozzarella cheese sticks.

Schedule Some "Me" Time When Visiting Family

Here's a way to reduce stress when visiting far-away family members that many of us often forget: Every now and again, find some alone time. Visit a mall. Go for a hike. See a historical site in a neighboring town. You'll find that you're less short-tempered with your relatives—and you'll have something new to talk about when Aunt Edna and Cousin Bobby start telling their same old jokes again.

whip it together! Crunchy Lime and Cayenne Pumpkin Seeds

These protein-rich snacks will keep for days. Their fiber is filling, and the B vitamins help your body metabolize carbohydrates.

In a small bowl, mix together 3 tablespoons fresh **lime juice**, ½ teaspoon **cayenne pepper**, ¼ teaspoon **salt**, and ⅛ teaspoon ground **black pepper**. Toast 1½ cups of raw **pumpkin seeds** in a dry skillet over medium heat for about 5 minutes, until lightly toasted. Pour lime mixture over pumpkin seeds and cook for 1 to 2 more minutes. Transfer to a zip-close bag and carry it with you in your purse or briefcase.

Put together a pocket-sized foot-care kit. When you're traveling, you want to see and do everything you can in a short time. But zipping from vista to landmark not only can wear out your feet, it can make you susceptible to "hot spots" and blisters. Although they seem innocent enough, blisters can lead to infections that can turn serious for someone with diabetes. To keep your feet feeling fine, fill a sandwich bag with several sheets of moleskin, several large and small adhesive bandages, and round-tipped bandage scissors. (If your pharmacy doesn't carry moleskin on the shelves, ask them to order it.) As soon as you feel a hot spot developing, cut off a piece of moleskin that's large enough to cover the spot and stick it on. If you discover a full-fledged blister, cover it with a bandage.

Wear lifesaving jewelry. No matter where your travels take you, you should always wear a medical alert bracelet or necklace to alert medical personnel to your diabetes status in the event of an emergency. One well-known company that provides alert jewelry and programs to inform health providers about your condition is MedicAlert, which you can find online at www.medicalert.org.

Step up your exercise with a pedometer. These are available at department stores and sporting goods stores. Many fitness experts recommend that you walk 10,000 steps a day, roughly equal to about five miles, to maintain good health. Clip your pedometer to your belt or waistband in the morning, and keep yourself moving until you've hit your goal for the day.

taking flight with confidence

In the early days of air travel, travelers looked at flying as a great adventure. Nowadays we often see it as a chore to endure before the *real* trip can begin. Here's how to ensure that your next flight will be safe and pleasant so you'll be all set and ready to go when the fun starts.

Bring your own meal or snack. These days, few airlines offer free meals; you're probably out of luck if you're flying economy class or you're on a relatively short flight. The meals and snacks that airlines do offer are not only expensive and unsatisfying, but unhealthy to boot. So tuck a turkey sandwich, pasta salad, an apple, or whole-wheat crackers and low-fat cheese into your carry-on bag along with some napkins and a plastic fork if you need one.

Book an aisle seat. You might be tempted to pity the person on the end of the row who has to get up whenever someone else wants to leave their seat. But that's the person who will arrive at his or her destination less cramped and more energized than anyone else, so seek out that seat, and use every opportunity to get up out of it. Sitting in a plane seat for hours on end raises the risk of deep vein thrombosis (DVT) or blood clots in the legs. Many factors often associated with diabetes—being overweight, being 60 or older, having poor blood circulation, and having a history of heart disease—are also linked to DVT, which can be life-threatening if the clot travels through the bloodstream and blocks blood flow to the lungs.

Set a digital reminder to get up. Time can easily get away from you while you're flying if you're sleeping or watching an in-flight movie. The next time you fly, wear a digital watch with an alarm, and set it to go off 60 or 90 minutes after takeoff. When the alarm goes off, stroll to the restroom and back, then reset your alarm to go off in another 60 or 90 minutes. Repeat this exercise throughout the flight.

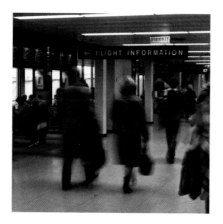

Use airport time to burn calories. Catching a plane involves a whole lot of hurry up and wait. While you're waiting for your plane to board, use that spare half-hour to tool around the terminal rather than grabbing an overpriced candy bar from the newsstand. If you combine the calories you'll burn moving your feet and the calories you save *not* chomping the chocolate, you'll end up a grand total of 420 calories behind where you would have been.

golden rule!   Bring Your Meds in Your Carry-On

Researchers from the University of Nebraska at Omaha and Wichita State University found that in 2006, major airlines mishandled an average of 6.5 baggage items per 1,000 passengers. That might not sound like many bags, but on a big jet that means two or three items of passengers' luggage will get misplaced. Some airlines have even worse baggage-handling ratings. Keep your diabetes supplies in a carry-on bag. If your checked suitcase gets lost on your next flight, it'll be the one containing your Hawaiian souvenirs, not your lifesaving medications. The temperature in the baggage bay is also very cold, which can affect your insulin.

Buy some bottled water once you've cleared security. Yes, the flight attendants on the plane will come around with the beverage cart once or twice, depending on the length of your flight, but you should drink more often than that to avoid dehydration, which can give you a headache and possibly raise your blood sugar. If you have to get up more often to use the bathroom, that's not a bad thing. Don't buy your water before you pass through security or you may be required to throw it out.

Ask at the gate for an exit row seat. These are seats you can only book once you're at the airport, and you can do it even if you already have a seat assignment—something not many people know. In an exit row you'll have oodles more room to stretch your legs.

Keep your feet on the move. To keep the blood flowing, do these simple foot exercises every half hour. With your heels on the floor, lift your toes up as far as possible. Hold for a few seconds, then release. Next, lift one foot slightly off the floor and draw circles in each direction with your toes. Repeat with the other foot. Finally, lift one heel as high as possible, keeping your toes on the floor. Repeat with the other foot.

For less stress, time your arrival at the airport just right. Nervous fliers can reduce their flight anxiety by leaving plenty of time to travel to the airport safely, park, check in with the agent, and get through security. Not leaving enough time to do these things will surely stress you out, which in turn will increase your blood glucose levels. For domestic flights on which you're checking a bag, arrive at the airport 90 minutes before the flight. For international flights, show up at least two hours before departure. Arrive 30 to 60 minutes earlier than that if you're flying during the holidays.

crash course

exercising with resistance bands

Packing fitness accessories that are lightweight, inexpensive, and portable can be your greatest motivation to exercise when you're away from home—and resistance bands are about as portable as you can get. Resistance bands are stretchy plastic bands used in strength-training exercises for your upper and lower body. Stretching the latex material provides resistance similar to the effect of weight lifting. Grasp the bands so that you feel challenged, rather than strained, by the resistance. Perform two or three sets of each of these resistance band exercises, doing 8 to 12 repetitions per set.

1 | biceps curl

Stand on the center of the resistance band with your feet hip-distance apart. **Grasp** an end of the band in each hand. Keep your arms down at your sides, palms facing forward.

Keeping your elbows at your sides, slowly **pull** your hands up to your shoulders and return them to the starting position.

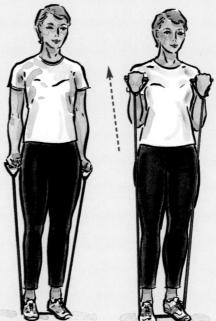

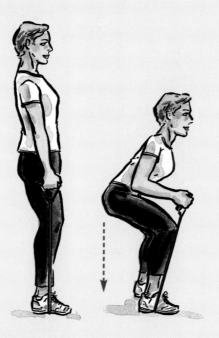

2 | squat

Stand on the center of the resistance band with your feet hip-distance apart. Grasp an end of the band in each hand. Start with your arms down at your sides, palms facing your body.

Bend at the waist and lower your backside into a squat, but not so far that your thighs are perpendicular to the floor. Keep your chest up, your back straight, and your toes farther forward than your knees. Now **push** with your legs to stand straight up, and then return to the squatting position.

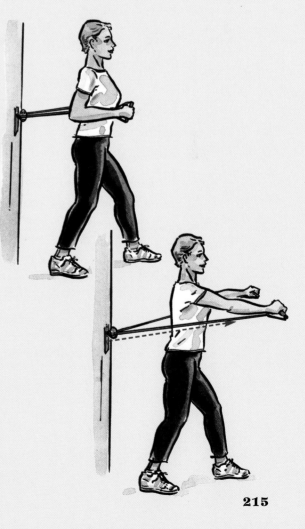

3 | arm extension

Start by securing the middle of the band around a fixed object (a door knob or banister, for instance). Face the center of the band and, for stability, **stand** with one foot a few inches farther forward than the other. Your knees should be bent slightly. **Grasp** an end of the resistance band in each hand. Hold your elbows at your sides, bent at right angles, with your hands in front of you and your palms facing down.

Slowly **push** your forearms down until your arms are straight and pointed toward the floor. Then return them to the starting position.

4 | chest press

Start by securing the middle of the band around a fixed object (a door knob or banister, for instance). Face away from the center of the band and, for stability, **stand** with one foot a few inches farther forward than the other and knees slightly bent. Hold an end of the band in each hand, and let the band run under your arms. Start with your hands slightly forward of your chest, forearms parallel to the ground and just below your shoulder.

Slowly **push** your arms forward until they are fully extended, keeping the hands shoulder-width apart, and then return to the starting position.

staying healthy while venturing abroad

Traveling to foreign countries offers many thrills: new customs, unusual foods, and exotic accents. But like any adventure it also poses potential challenges. Before you depart for distant shores, take a few easy steps to help ensure a safe, fun trip.

Get your shots early. Book an appointment with your doctor six to eight weeks before your trip. Ask her whether you'll need any vaccinations to get into the country you're visiting, and get those taken care of as soon as possible. Some take weeks to take effect.

Call your health insurance company a month ahead of time. Know before you go what medical expenses your health insurance company covers while you travel internationally and what they don't. If they don't offer the coverage you think you need, consider purchasing supplemental traveler's insurance.

Find a doc abroad before you leave home. Make a list of doctors who speak your language and pack it in your carry-on bag. English speakers can get a list of doctors from the International Association for Medical Assistance to Travellers (www.iamat.org). It's also helpful to bring the contact information for your government's consulate serving the area you'll be visiting in case you find yourself in need of help. They may be able to assist you in finding a doctor who speaks your language.

Learn a few key terms in the native tongue. Talking to locals in their language, even if it's just to say "hello" or "have a nice day," makes your interactions more fun. Buy a phrase book, and while you're studying it, make a list of other phrases that might come in handy, such as, "I have diabetes," "My blood sugar is low," or "I need orange juice." Leave three lines in your notebook for each phrase that you write down: On the top line, write the phrase in English. On the second line, write it in the foreign language. On the third line, spell it out phonetically. This way, you should be able to pronounce it yourself, but if you can't make the person understand, you can just point to the translated version.

Research the local cuisine. Other cultures' cuisines may include unfamiliar foods and dishes with strange ingredients. While you're reading about your destination, bone up on the local specialties. Seek out appetizers, entrées, and desserts that will work well with your eating plan, and practice saying the names of these foods (or write them down on "cheat sheets" you can take to the restaurant) so you'll remember them.

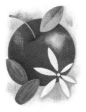

Teach yourself phrases that might come in handy, such as, "I need orange juice."

getting quality rest during hotel stays

Let's face it, few people sleep as well in hotel rooms as they do at home. But quality sleep is key to enjoying the next day and to keeping your blood sugar on an even keel.

Book a quiet room in advance. Shouting, music, and mysterious clangs at night leave you stressed and tired the next day. Ask for a room away from the elevator, vending machine, and ice machine, without much foot traffic nearby. You'll also want plenty of floors between you and any wedding parties, student groups, or other gatherings.

Bring a few comforting items from home. Packing your own pillow and your favorite pajamas, along with other calming items—the book that you read before turning in or the needlework you do for winding down—will help you feel more comfortable and sleep better in your new surroundings.

Inspect your quarters carefully before turning in. After you've brushed your teeth, take a quick turn about your hotel room and make sure the curtains are tightly drawn, the air conditioner or heater is set to a comfortable temperature, and the door is locked. Also check the clock radio and make sure the alarm is turned off (or set it to the time *you* want to get up).

Block out the outside world. Pack earplugs and a sleep mask and don them before putting your head on the pillow.

Request a wake-up call from the hotel operator. Why is it that the clock radios in hotel rooms always seem so much more complicated than the ones we have at home? Stop worrying about whether the alarm will go off at 7 a.m. or 7 p.m., and have the front-desk operator give you a ring when it's time to rise and shine.

golden rule! Check Your Feet at the End of Every Day

It's tempting when you get back to your hotel room after a long day on your feet to slip off your shoes, fall back on the bed, and relax. Just be sure to add one step to that routine. Every time you remove your shoes while you're on vacation, check your feet for red spots, blisters, irritation, cuts, or nail injuries. Treat any foot problems according to your doctor's recommendations. Your feet can take a pounding when you're seeing the sights, and troubles with your tootsies can cause health complications long after your vacation is over.

work exercise into your time away

Whether you're traveling for business or pleasure, odds are you'll be sitting for long periods on your way to your destination, and when you get there, you'll probably eat more than you should. Plan to counteract the effects of idleness and overindulgence by getting around on some good old-fashioned foot power during your stay.

Zero in on the area's best parks, zoos, and gardens. Whether you're going away for an extended vacation or just a weekend, order a visitor's packet from your destination's chamber of commerce or the destination itself and scan through it for attractions to visit that involve plenty of walking or other exercise, such as nature preserves, parks, gardens, and museums. You'd be amazed how many miles you can log spending a fun, relaxing afternoon gawking at the animals in the zoo.

See the sights on two wheels. Ask your travel agent about guided bicycle tours in the city you'll be visiting—or search for the words "bicycle tours" plus the city of your choice on the Internet. You're not going to find a much better way to enjoy the sights of a city than on a bike. Unlike taxi or bus tours, you can see attractions at a slower pace, and you can smell, touch, and savor your surroundings. And unlike walking, you can easily see miles of attractions in a few hours without suffering from sore feet.

Take a stroll through the town square. Visiting the social hub of a town or city is the surest way to absorb the local flavor, and it's even more enjoyable when you make the stroll arm-in-arm with your partner. Together you'll be able to size up restaurants for tonight's dinner, pick up souvenirs at shops, and meet locals who can give you insiders' advice on must-see attractions.

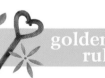

golden rule! Wear Plenty of Sunscreen

After being cooped up indoors most of the year, it's natural to seek out the sun on vacation. But some diabetes drugs, such as glipizide (Glucotrol) and glyburide (Diabeta), can make your skin especially sensitive to sunlight. And a bad sunburn can raise your blood sugar and even lead to infection. Use a sunscreen with an SPF of 30 or higher, and put it on much more liberally than you think you should—studies show most people don't use nearly enough and don't reapply often enough. If you have trouble reaching your legs and feet while applying sunscreen, ask a travel companion to do it for you, or buy the spray-on kind to make the task easier.

Be an early bird. If your trip includes a visit to an amusement park, zoo, or boardwalk, arrive the minute it opens. The place may be much less crowded, and you'll be able to spend your time seeing and doing what you came for rather than standing in line getting sore feet and a sunburn. If the place you want to visit is crowded in the mornings (call ahead and ask if you're not sure), try late afternoon.

Hula, tango, and fish like the locals do. You know the old saying: "When in Rome, do as the Romans do." Well, if you're in Argentina, take a tango lesson. In Hawaii, learn to hula. Wherever your travels may take you, there's an activity that will help you learn more about the area and its people—and keep you moving in the process.

Send yourself on a hunt for great photos. Before you head off on your trip, make a wish list of at least 25 photos that you'd love to snap during your vacation. Options on your checklist might include birds or wildlife in their natural setting; a self-portrait at a cathedral or fortress; a sunrise; a landscape with no cars, roads, or billboards in the picture; and a panoramic shot taken from a high vantage point. Be sure to give yourself an ambitious list that requires walking all over town to get the shots you want. Reward yourself for achieving your goal by purchasing a beautiful photo album in which to display your photos.

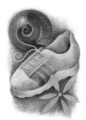

Diabetes can make it harder for the body to cool itself.

Hit the museums during the midday heat peak. Even if you're vigilant about using sunscreen, it's smart to move inside during the hottest hours— usually between noon and 2 p.m.—to ensure that you don't overheat or get a sunburn. Diabetes may cause your sunburn to heal more slowly or lead to infection, and it may be harder for people with diabetes to cool themselves. Use these hours to see a museum exhibit, grab a bite to eat, or take a scenic trip by car or covered boat.

Keep a duffel bag packed with workout gear. If you travel frequently for business, stuff a small backpack or duffel bag with all the workout gear you need, and keep it under your bed at home so it's always ready to go. Include sneakers, shorts, socks, shirt, jog bra, swimsuit, pedometer, towel, soap, deodorant, and a combination lock. You'll be able to squeeze in a quick jog or walk at your hotel when you arrive, or use an airport gym during a layover. You'll also have the gear you need to clean up afterward.

Hit the gym or walking trail first thing in the morning. Business travel is filled with meetings, conferences, interviews, and meals with clients. If you don't make time for physical activity, it won't happen. Getting it in first thing in the morning is the best time for many travelers: Your schedule is least likely to be hectic then, and the vigor of a morning workout can keep you going the rest of the day.

staying healthy on the high seas

For many people a cruise is a dream come true—a floating paradise, the ultimate luxury. And despite the pitfalls of the all-you-can-eat buffets, the truth is, cruise vacations can be just as healthy and active as you want them to be. So pack your sneakers, your swimsuit, and your dancing shoes, and follow these tips. You'll return from your vacation in shipshape!

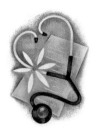

Keep a bottle of hand sanitizer in your pocket

Aim to burn more calories than you do at home. This should be simple—you can easily fit in at least 30 minutes of walking during the average shore excursion. And on a moderate-size ship, you can log a mile with just four laps around the promenade deck, which is designed for just that (no deck chairs in the way). That's not even counting the exercise you can do in the swimming pool, in the gym, or in the ocean (snorkeling anyone?).

Call ahead for a sample menu, or find one online. Bring it to your dietitian, who can help you figure out how to make choices that will fit into your eating plan, so you're not overwhelmed when you get there.

Pick out one "prize" at the buffet table. From the outside, a cruise liner looks like a ship. Once you're on board, it looks more like a floating smorgasbord. Before you fill your plate, eyeball the entire buffet table and choose one small, indulgent item as a treat to yourself, so you, too, can feel as if you've been part of the fun, without going "overboard."

Give germs the rub-out. It's easy to pick up a stomach virus on a cruise ship. Feeling nauseous not only ruins your day, it'll make controlling your blood sugar much more difficult. The solution is literally at your fingertips: Wash your hands frequently. Do it after you touch items that other passengers frequently touch and right before meals. For extra protection, keep a bottle of hand sanitizer in your pocket and use it right before your food arrives. You'll kill off any germs you picked up opening the dining-room door.

Sign up for the active stuff. Some shore excursions, like eating at a famous local restaurant or seeing sites by bus, barely require getting up off your backside. But others, like biking excursions or snorkeling trips, provide a great workout. Some cruises even let you prebook shore excursions. Just make sure that you choose ones that are a good match for your physical abilities. If you have any doubts, talk to the activities director.

While ashore, choose your food carefully (or bring your own). The food on cruise ships is usually safe, but depending on what country you're in, the same isn't necessarily true when you venture ashore. Avoid raw fruits and vegetables, tap water, iced beverages, and food sold by street vendors.

chapter thirteen

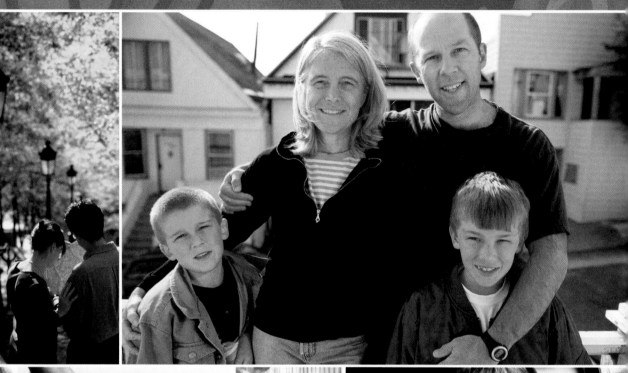

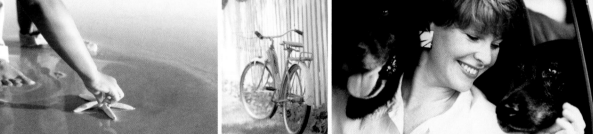

in your family

Your diabetes affects your family, too: If *you* have to live with
the disease for the rest of your life, so do they. Here's how to get
the support you need while keeping family life happy,
active, and stress free.

bring your family on board

The more your family knows about diabetes, the more they'll appreciate what you're going through as you try to manage your health and the more they'll be able to help. You should never feel like you're in this alone.

Don't hide your diabetes. Some patients try to avoid informing their spouses of their diagnosis, partly out of a stoic "I can handle it alone" attitude. The truth is, managing diabetes affects so many aspects of your life that you need the cooperation and understanding of everyone under your roof.

Bring home literature about diabetes management. You may know this information because you *have* diabetes, but someone who doesn't might forget about some of the issues—such as the need to check blood sugar levels several times a day, to eat at regular intervals, and to watch calories and carbs—that you cope with every day.

Bring loved ones to your diabetes support group. Letting your spouse or family members listen in will give them an excellent window on what you're facing now and the challenges you might encounter later. They may even pick up some tips that will help you.

If you need help from your spouse, ask. Many couples have problems communicating their wants and needs. For instance, it's common for women to think: "If my husband won't help with the housekeeping, why would he want to help me with my diabetes?" Don't brood. Tell your spouse what you need. Perhaps it's time to exercise, or Thursdays off from cooking. You might be surprised how willingly your spouse will help.

Train your family to recognize and treat low blood sugar. Everyone in your household should know the signs—rapid heartbeat, sweating, double vision, mental confusion—and how to take emergency measures. (The first thing they should know? That people who are hypoglycemic usually claim to feel fine when they're not.) Your family will need to know where you store your emergency foods and how much to give you. If you have a prescription for glucagon, train your family to inject it.

Teach them about high blood sugar, too. They should know the symptoms—unusual thirst, the need to urinate frequently, blurry vision, and reduced energy—and be ready to take emergency measures. Make sure they know how to test your blood sugar, and if you're on insulin, how and when to administer it.

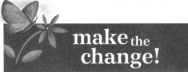

make the change!

The habit: Involving your family in your healthy habits.

The result: They'll be less likely to develop diabetes.

The proof: A major study called the Diabetes Prevention Program, which involved more than 3,000 people with prediabetes—most of whom were obese and had a family history of the disease—showed they could reduce their risk of developing full-blown diabetes by 58 percent by modifying their lifestyles. The study participants accomplished this by switching to a healthful diet and getting 30 minutes of moderate physical activity on five days out of each week.

food and family

If you and your spouse are used to sitting down to big steak dinners or weekly fast-food meals, at least one of you is going to have to change your ways. Your family members need to realize right off the bat that you're serious about following your new eating plan. Why not get them to join you? Remember, the same habits that you're aiming for—eating well and exercising regularly—are good for just about everybody.

Eat meals together as a family. Experts say that families reap enormous emotional benefits when its members regularly eat meals together: Family communication is better, people eat more nutritiously, and the behavior of children is better overall. All of this means that your household is less a den of stress than a harmonious oasis.

Make your own healthful selections at the supermarket. If you aren't the primary grocery shopper for the family, hit the supermarket with your spouse and make sure that the shopping cart contains foods that you like that also fit into your eating plan. This will increase the odds that home-cooked meals are appealing to you and help you reach your goals for weight loss and blood sugar control. It also will reduce the chances of arguments cropping up over menu selection.

Downsize—don't eliminate—the junk food in your cupboard. Unless you do all of the household food shopping, you may feel as if you don't have much control over whether tempting foods enter your house. On the other hand, you might also be reluctant to ban all junk foods and "punish" your family. There is a middle ground: Ask the family shopper to buy those tempting foods in smaller sizes—half of a cake instead of a whole one, for instance, small containers of ice cream, and small bags of potato chips. If you end up indulging in these items, you'll at least have some automatic portion control.

Create a playbook of healthful recipe favorites. Ask each person in your household to scour cookbooks, food magazines, and the Internet for healthful recipes that look appealing. Try them out and put the "keepers" in your recipe file. Teach every family member how to make these meals—or at least the ones that they chose—so the daily cooking duties don't just fall on one person. The more involved (and proud) your family members are of their cooking contributions, the more fun healthy eating will be.

Flank less-healthy entrées with bowls of veggies. On a night when the main dish at dinner does not fit with your meal plan, set a large bowl of raw or steamed vegetables on the table as a side dish. Take just a small portion of the entrée and extra helpings of the vegetable. Other members of your family probably won't be as meticulous about healthful eating as you, but that's okay. When you show this kind of flexibility, everyone will be satisfied by the household's dinner fare over the long haul.

Start a compost pile. Many families have a "clean your plate" rule that just encourages everyone to overeat. However, when there's an Earth-friendly way to recycle excess food, leaving food on your plate will not seem so wasteful. Plant-based table scraps and the trimmings from fruits and vegetables go in the pile. Turning your compost pile with a shovel once a week and dumping in your grass clippings will add a little more physical activity to your life as well.

When schedules conflict, adjust your eating. Say your grandson is playing his big clarinet solo in a talent show at noon, right when you should be having lunch. Why not pack your meal in a refrigerated lunch bag? To hold you over during the performance, eat half of your sandwich during the car ride to the show, and eat the rest of your lunch as soon as it's over.

whip it together! Seared Cod in Zesty Herb and Tomato Sauce

Getting finicky families to eat fish isn't easy, but this zesty dish made with mild-tasting cod is one almost anyone can love.

4 (4-ounce) **cod** filets (1-inch thick)

Salt and **pepper**

2 teaspoons **olive oil**

1 chopped medium **onion**

2 **garlic** cloves

2 cans (14 ounces each) **diced tomatoes** with Italian herbs

2 tablespoons **tomato paste**

2 tablespoons **balsamic vinegar** or ¼ cup **dry red wine**

2 tablespoons minced fresh **basil**

2 teaspoons minced fresh **oregano**

Sprinkle the cod filets lightly with salt and pepper. Heat the olive oil in a large skillet over medium heat. Add the cod and sauté on both sides until lightly browned, about 8 to 10 minutes. Remove the fish from the pan. Add the onion and garlic. Sauté for 2 minutes. Add the diced tomatoes and tomato paste and bring to a boil. Lower the heat and add the balsamic vinegar or red wine. Simmer over low heat for 20 minutes. Add the basil and oregano. Simmer for 3 minutes. Serve the fish topped with the tomato sauce.

defuse and de-stress

The fact that you have diabetes can be stressful for everyone around you. The people who love you may worry—too much, sometimes—and the time and expense of taking good care of yourself my throw a wrench in the normal family budget or schedule. Take these simple steps to keep conflict under control.

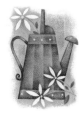

Get your spouse on board with your health goals for maximum support.

Allay family fears with education and frank talk. It's not uncommon to find that a close relation of a person with diabetes is more worried about the disease than the patient himself. The sources of such fears are often lack of knowledge and misconceptions about diabetes. Explain carefully what diabetes is and what you do to manage the disease. Share pertinent books and pamphlets and, if you are explaining diabetes to a child, use age-appropriate language. A child will probably become more at ease about your diabetes if you discuss it a little at a time in incidental conversations rather than in one long conversation.

Clarify your spouse's role at medical appointments. Decide whether you want your spouse to accompany you to medical appointments, and make sure this understanding is clear between the two of you. You may prefer to discuss your diabetes alone with your doctor. On the other hand, it often helps to have an ally in the examination room to ask questions you didn't think of and to make sure that instructions are clear. When your spouse understands his or her role in your medical appointments, there will be less frustration and stress between you.

Budget for your medical expenses. When you write up your monthly household budget, make sure that you factor in medical expenses like testing gear and diabetes medications. Money problems are the most common causes of marital problems—and divorce. The more realistic and upfront you can be with your spouse about the effect that your condition will have on your bottom line, the better.

Work with your spouse to establish health goals. Remember, your spouse has a vested interested in keeping you healthy. Decide together what efforts you'll make to better manage your disease, such as a daily 30-minute walk after dinner or bringing lunch from home. When the two of you set these goals jointly, your efforts to manage your disease will be less likely to spawn resentment or arguments. For instance, you might decide that you will start taking a salad to work every day for lunch. If your spouse is "on board" with this idea, he or she might make sure that fresh salad ingredients are available, might find special containers that make carrying them easier, or might help prepare these salads in the evenings.

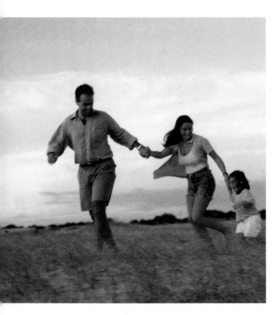

Feeling nagged? Make a date with the Diabetes Police. Family members who constantly offer unsought advice or lecture you about how you should take care of your health, can drive you batty or just shut you down. Instead of ignoring the problem (especially if you are living with that person), invite them out for a casual lunch or dinner. Being in public can help keep tempers from flaring. Calmly explain how much you love them, and tell them that you appreciate their concern. Then let them know what you would find helpful, as well as what isn't helpful. Be as honest and open as possible. You may want to write down your thoughts ahead of time, so you're sure to get all your points covered.

Declare a moratorium on shouting, profanity, hurtful words, and talking through clenched teeth. At a time when tempers are cool, talk to your family about the direct connection between hostility and health. Anger and stress prompt your body to release hormones that drive blood sugar levels up. If you're the grumpy one, check to see if your behavior is due to low blood sugar levels. Maybe talking after a meal is a better idea.

Make stress-relieving "dates" with yourself. Lower your own stress levels, and the family's will follow. It's equally important whether you're a workaholic or you're retired to find outlets for stress and for boredom, which can cause their own kinds of stress. Whether it's evening walks, knitting, reading, or going to yoga class, make the time, then follow through. You'll be better able to treat conflicts that do arise with calmness and compassion.

Put your marriage first. A growing pile of research links unhappy marriages with high blood pressure, high levels of stress hormones, and depression. Help yours along by remembering to say "thank you" to your spouse at least once a day and offering to do small kindnesses without being asked. If you marriage is really in trouble, see a marriage counselor.

surviving holidays and special occasions

Family celebrations are supposed to be welcome distractions from everyday cares. But for someone with diabetes, they can make "everyday cares" bigger problems than they already are. With holidays come fatty, high-carb feasts, irregular eating schedules, and plenty of family stress to go around. Take a few of the following steps to make holidays gatherings what they should be: fun.

Stock the freezer with healthy meals. Everyone's overly busy during the holidays, and most of us want to spend our time shopping, decorating, or seeing friends and family, which leaves less time to cook healthy meals. Take defensive action several weeks ahead of time by cooking meals intended specifically for the freezer. You'll be thankful later when you can pop one of the meals into the oven or microwave and turn your attention instead to writing out holiday cards with a personal message in each.

Win the food-pushing relative over to your point of view. Many of us have a pushy cousin, uncle, or mother-in-law who never seems satisfied unless you have had several helpings of their signature dish. How on earth can you defend yourself from their entreaties? If they won't accept a simple "No, thank you," bring out the big guns. Confess that you just can't resist their prize-winning pie, but that your doctor and nutritionist insist that you show some restraint. If you relent, take a small serving, then ask for their help—in front of others—in resisting seconds. They will quickly come to your aid, lest they be thought of as saboteurs.

Refuse food with a smile and a compliment. When you must decline food that a relative or friend has lovingly prepared, make it clear to the cook or baker that you are not rejecting her—you are just sidestepping a

golden rule!   Keep the Focus on Fun, Not Food

Most holidays are associated with certain foods (the Fourth of July practically dictates burgers and hot dogs, and Christmas at your house might not be the same without your aunt's green been casserole), but that doesn't mean food has to be the main focus. Instead, throw yourself into the other rituals a holiday brings, whether it's birthday presents, fireworks, costumes, caroling, tree trimming, dying Easter eggs, or writing a love note to your Valentine.

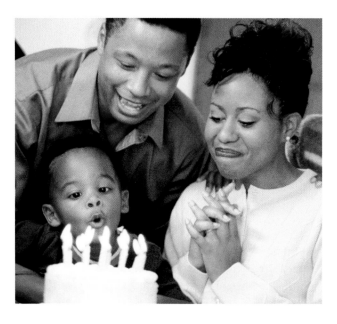

food that doesn't fit into your meal plan. How can you keep from hurting her feelings? Say "no thanks" wistfully, then tell her how delicious her cake looks. You might even tell her you'd love to pass the recipe along to a friend who loves coconut cake, or ask questions about her cake-decorating technique. She'll soon be so flattered that she'll forget you haven't had a bite!

Modify your eating times so that they jive with your relatives'. Do your in-laws' meal schedules fly in the face of yours? Here's how to compromise: Say they wake up later than you do and serve a late breakfast at 10:30. Then they skip lunch and serve Christmas "dinner" at 3 p.m. To keep your blood sugar steady without overdoing it on calories, have an early-morning snack (such as a piece of whole-grain toast) before your relatives rise and shine. Their late breakfast will count as your "real" breakfast, plus some of your lunch. Enjoy the 3 p.m. meal—but don't overdo it!—and have a small snack at around 8 p.m. Be sure to pack your monitoring equipment so that you can see how this work-around plan is affecting your blood sugar.

Get the family on its feet. Walk about the neighborhood caroling; get all family members involved in decorating the house; or find out where the most elaborately decorated houses in town are and trek out there (with some sugar-free cocoa in your thermos). Remember that exercise is the perfect antidote for a buttery dinner roll or piece of pie.

Cut down your own Christmas tree. Rather than buying a tree from a roadside lot where the trees have been drying out for weeks, visit a tree farm that allows you to cut your own. It will be fresher and probably less expensive than they are at the lot. You'll burn off calories and combat some of the blood-sugar effects of the sugar cookie you snuck by traipsing around the grounds in search of just the right tree. And your family will have one more fond holiday memory to look back on.

Indulge in only the most special holiday treats. Skip the candy corn at Halloween, the frozen pumpkin pie at Thanksgiving, and the store-bought cookies at Christmas, but do save some calories in your "budget" to sample treats that are homemade and special to your family, such as your wife's special Yule log cake. Training yourself what to indulge in and what to skip is much like budgeting your mad money: Do you want to blow it on garbage that you can buy anywhere or on a very special, one-of-a-kind souvenir? Just don't completely deprive yourself on festive days—your willpower will eventually snap, and you'll end up overeating.

Have pumpkin soup instead of pumpkin pie. If you're doing your best not to over-indulge in sugary, high-carb treats, but you still want to enjoy the classic tastes of fall, look to pumpkin soup instead of pumpkin pie or cookies and to baked apples with cinnamon and a touch of brown sugar rather than apple pie a la mode.

Choose between a slice of pie and a scoop of mashed potatoes. If you know your favorite pie is being served for dessert, make a decision: Do you want to spend your meal's carb allowance there or on the stuffing or mashed potatoes at the table? Of course, under normal circumstances, you should favor dinner food over dessert, but if it's a special day and you know you can't resist a small slice of dessert, just make sure you account for the carbs and calories by cutting back elsewhere.

Bring a tray of beautifully arranged veggies or fruit to the party. Even if you weren't asked to bring anything to your neighbor's New Year's bash, don't go empty-handed. Prepare a platter that's piled high with your favorite fresh fruits and/or veggies, along with a low-calorie, low-fat dip. Munch on these before or during dinner, and you'll be less tempted to fill up on foods that will blow your calorie budget.

Offer to bring a dessert. Find a delicious recipe that's low in carbs and calories, and present it proudly. That way, you'll know there will be one dessert at the gathering that you can safely eat.

Pour the gravy and sauces lightly. You may not be able to control what's being served at a holiday meal, but you can make the turkey, roast beef, and even mashed potatoes and stuffing much healthier by foregoing the sauce or gravy or spooning on just a small amount.

Make your turkey white. Turkey breast is one of the leanest meats you'll find. Just stick to the breast, not the dark meat (legs and thighs), which is considerably higher in calories and fat. And always say no to the skin!

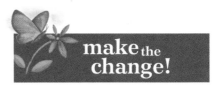

make the change!

The habit: Staying physically active during the holidays.

The result: Gaining less weight over the years.

The proof: A study conducted by the U.S. government found adults gained, on average, more than a pound of body weight during the winter holidays—and that they were not at all likely to shed that weight the following year. (That may not sound like a lot now, but it means having to buy roomier pants after a few Christmases pass.) The good news is that the people who reported the most physical activity through the holiday season showed the least weight gain. Some even managed to lose weight.

whip it together! Happy Birthday Frozen Yogurt Cake

The best part about celebrating a birthday isn't blowing out the candles—it's digging in to cake and ice cream. This recipe delivers both, with less fat and calories.

Prepare a 20-ounce box of reduced-fat **brownie mix** according to package directions, and pour into two 8-inch round cake pans that have been lined with wax paper. Bake according to package directions. Remove the cake from the oven and cool in the pan for 10 minutes. Turn out onto cooling racks, remove the waxed paper, and let cool. When cool, place one layer on a work surface. Spread with 1 quart "no-sugar-added" **frozen yogurt** and 2 cups sliced **strawberries**. Top with the remaining cake layer. Wrap loosely in foil and freeze for 3 hours. When ready to serve, remove from the freezer and let stand for 5 to 6 minutes. Drizzle with sugar-free **chocolate syrup**, if desired. Slice into 1-inch pieces.

Add turkey or chicken to those backyard burgers. If your family hosts an annual backyard bash, make less-fattening burgers by kneading ground turkey or chicken in with the beef. Few people will know the difference, but your arteries sure will.

Toast the New Year with just one glass of bubbly. You may be celebrating, but that doesn't mean that that you should send your meal plan (and your judgment) on holiday. Alcohol can interfere with your blood sugar by slowing the release of glucose into the bloodstream; it also contain a lot of calories—89 calories per glass of white wine or champagne, 55 calories in a shot of vodka, and 170 calories in a pint of stout beer. What's more, alcohol breaks down your inhibitions and judgment, which makes you that much less likely to resist the junk foods that you would otherwise be able to pass up.

Check your blood sugar more often. Despite your very best intentions, you may be eating more, or differently, than you do the rest of the year. If you're dining at the home of friends or relatives, you may not be able to accurately estimate the amount of carbohydrate you're eating or know how the foods on the table will affect your blood sugar, so it's especially important to check your blood sugar regularly, especially after eating. Remember, general guidelines state that glucose levels should be between 90 and 130 mg/dl before meals, less than 180 mg/dl two hours after starting a meal, and less than 140 mg/dl at bedtime.

ramp up physical activity as a family

Being the only member of the household who exercises is like, well, swimming upstream. But if you make physical activity part of your family's culture, everyone will benefit. If you have kids in your household, remember that they follow your lead. In fact, studies show that family environment is one of the strongest predictors of childhood obesity. If you have grandkids who visit regularly, be sure to include them in the fun, too.

Start a new family ritual. Take an after-dinner walk to the frozen yogurt parlor every Wednesday or a family bike ride on the first Sunday of the month. Soon enough it will become second nature to everyone—and something the whole family looks forward to.

Pick your own produce. Rally the troops, or at least grab your spouse, and spend an early weekend morning gathering berries at a "pick-your-own" farm. You'll get fresher berries along with your fresh air and exercise. And at home, you can all enjoy the "fruits" of you labor.

Repair or replace worn exercise gear. Nothing sidetracks a family bike ride faster than a flat tire or a loose chain. And backyard or driveway ball games fizzle fast when the ball's deflated. Make it a point to keep your equipment in working order—that also means sharpening ice skates and restringing tennis rackets—and there will be one less barrier to keeping your family moving. Maintaining equipment properly can even prevent accidents.

Take the wife and kids for roller-skating lessons. Has it been a while since you've been on wheels? Call the local roller rink and sign your family up for skating lessons. Believe it or not, roller-skating is pretty good aerobic exercise, and it's a fun group activity that your family can participate in year round. It's particularly fun if you ask the DJ to play your favorite tunes, and boogie together in a conga line. Once you feel confident enough on eight wheels, go for a spin outside—just be careful on those hills!

Chart your expeditions. Here's a sure way to get your spouse and kids excited about active exploring: In your family room, post a map that covers the areas in which your family typically vacations. "Collect" mountains, lakes, rivers, trails, and other geographical features by hiking, climbing, or boating there during family trips. Record these "conquests" by marking them on the map with pushpins. On subsequent trips, family members will want to get out of the car and experience nature firsthand so that they can add pushpins to the map back home.

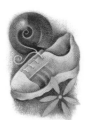

Keeping your exercise equipment in working order will help keep your family moving.

Give your two legs to a good cause. Watch the local newspaper and community bulletin boards for announcements about fund-raising events that'll make you get off your duff for charity—like walk-a-thons or five-kilometer races—and participate in such events as a family. Choose charities that are meaningful to your family. For example, you might honor your mother's battle with breast cancer by walking in her memory and wearing family T-shirts emblazoned with her photograph. Not only will you benefit from the exercise, but you'll also create new social connections, feel good about helping worthy causes, and tell your favorite anecdotes about Mom as you go.

Sign up for an "Adopt a Street" program. Many community groups such as churches and service organizations strike an arrangement with local governments in which they "adopt" certain sections of roadway. Several times a year, these groups will organize crews to pick up litter along the roadside, bag it up, and deposit it at a trash collection site. If you need some relief in the middle of the litter collecting, take a turn as the flag person who warns oncoming cars of the road crew ahead.

Encourage the grandkids to join active programs. If you have children in the house or grandchildren nearby, help them develop an interest in organized sports or in clubs, such as the Boy or Girl Scouts, that involve physical activity. When the youngsters you're close to are active, you inevitably will become more active, too. How could you not, if you're helping Junior practice his Little League pitches, or your little Brownie Scout needs someone to accompany her on nature walks and help her identify plants to get her next merit badge?

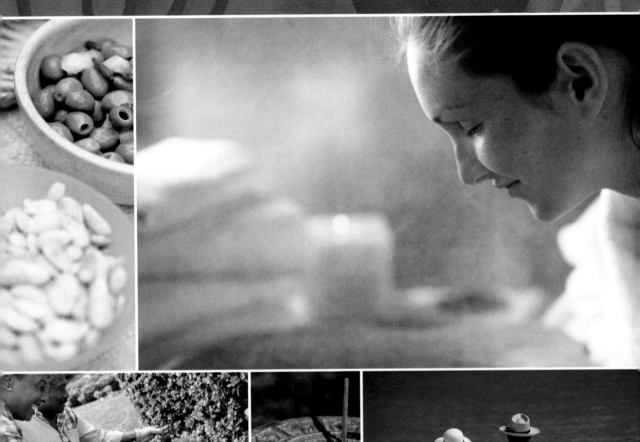

chapter fourteen

in your mind

Diabetes may be a physical problem, but beating the disease
is just as much about what goes on in your head as what goes on
in your body. As with so many things, a positive
mind-set makes all the difference.

success starts in your head

If you were managing a business, you'd expect highs and lows, successes and setbacks. Managing diabetes is no different—except there are no vacations from it. You'll want to set goals, expect the occasional down day, and above all, believe you can succeed at keeping your blood sugar under control, the key to avoiding some very serious and sometimes irreversible health consequences. Having a positive outlook has even been shown to reduce stress, improve mood, boost immune system functioning, and lower the risk of heart disease. The best news? You don't have to be a born Pollyanna (and most people aren't) to adopt a winning attitude.

Choose to fight. When people are diagnosed with a life-threatening form of cancer, some choose to fight, while others choose to give up. Being diagnosed with diabetes, even though it's hardly a death sentence, is a little similar. If you had a close relative who suffered serious complications from diabetes, you might throw your hands up and assume you're going to suffer the same fate. Or you could take the attitude "That isn't going to happen to me." The choice is yours. Just remember, there is no good reason to give up. Diabetes is very manageable, and most aspects of managing it are under your direct control.

Visualize success. There are no two ways about it: Taking good care of your diabetes requires some determination. Using imagery can help. Sit down and close your eyes. Visualize what you want to see yourself doing in the future. Do you want to be alive and healthy enough to play with your grandchildren as they grow up? Do you want to retire to a lifestyle in which you're not limited by health problems, so you can enjoy golfing, fishing, traveling, or whatever you love? Thinking about your dreams and aspirations for tomorrow can help stoke the fire under your motivation today.

Think of yourself as a person *with* diabetes, not as a diabetic. According to psychologist Mary Cerreto, PhD, "If you think of yourself as a diabetic, what comes first? Being a diabetic. Instead, if you say, 'I'm a person with diabetes,' then diabetes is just *part* of your life, not the whole thing." View having diabetes as you would being nearsighted: It's something you need to account for, but it certainly doesn't define you.

Make a list of goals and update it once a month. Start with three specific, clear, short-term measures. If

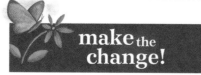

make the change!

The habit: Telling yourself you can do it.

The result: Better diabetes control.

The proof: When Denver Veterans Affairs Medical Center researchers recorded the mindsets of 88 people with diabetes and then followed them for a year, they found that those who reported a strong belief in their ability to take care of their diabetes were more likely to follow their diet and exercise recommendations and had lower blood sugar, compared to people who reported low confidence.

Accept That You Have Diabetes for Life

golden rule!

You've probably heard of the Serenity Prayer: "God grant me the serenity to accept the things I cannot change, the courage to change the things I can, and the wisdom to know the difference." This prayer about acceptance is a great reminder that some parts of our lives are not in our control, but others are. For instance, you can't change the fact that you have diabetes, but you can find the courage to alter your lifestyle in ways that will help you control your diabetes better. When you're feeling worried, sad, or irritable, stop and say this little prayer. Afterward, ask yourself what you need to accept and what you can change.

you just received your diagnosis, taking your meds on time and checking your blood sugar when you're supposed to might be enough for you to deal with at first. Once you feel like you're used to your routine, you can add another goal, such as eating five fruits and veggies per day, or taking a 30-minute walk three days a week. Specific, realistic, and limited goals will keep you from getting overwhelmed.

Stop dwelling on "poor me." Almost everyone has at least one major problem to deal with in life, be it a health problem, a financial challenge, or marital trouble. If you catch yourself having a pity party because of your diabetes, remind yourself that no one's life is perfect. Then take a few minutes to remind yourself of the future you've visualized, and tell yourself that it's up to you to make it happen by eating healthy, staying active, and monitoring your blood sugar (and acting on the results).

Spend 10 minutes in the morning contemplating the day ahead. Sit with your cup of coffee, tea, or juice, and set positive and conscious intentions for how you want your day to go and what you'll need to do to make sure it happens. Do you have your medications organized and your monitor ready to go? When will you fit in your daily walk? If you haven't packed a healthy lunch, what's your game plan for buying one? If you have a hectic day ahead, think about specific strategies you'll use to help you stay calm, such as deep breathing. Remember that keeping your stress levels in check will help you manage your blood sugar better. You can write down your thoughts and answers, just think about them, or pray to a higher power to help you succeed.

Get in the habit of giving thanks. Before you get out of bed in the morning, prior to eating a meal, and when you're preparing to go to bed, take a moment to appreciate the things you might typically take for granted, such as having shelter, regular meals, clean water, clothes, and friends. And don't forget to be grateful for access to health insurance, top-rate medications, and the ability to improve your well-being with diet and exercise. Counting your blessings will make you more aware of how lucky you really are.

Say "no" to your inner skeptic. When a "downer" thought threatens to drag you into the deep, fight back. If you find yourself thinking that you'll never lose weight or get your blood sugar under control, tell yourself "no!" in your firmest, most commanding voice, whether you do it in your head or out loud. Sometimes this is all it takes to stop nagging, negative thoughts from snowballing into a defeatist attitude.

Now think again. Once you've successfully stalled a negative thought, it's time to put something more positive in its place. If you were thinking along the lines of, "I'll never change," or "I'll always be sick," try to be more objective, specific, and fair with yourself. Are there other ways for you to look at the situation? For example, "I'm feeling lousy right now. Maybe my blood sugar is low. I'll check it and see if I should have a snack."

What's Your Mind-Set?

Having a can-do attitude starts with being willing to make some changes in your life to improve your health. But being diagnosed with a chronic disease like diabetes can send a person through a series of emotions similar to the stages of grief. It's not a linear process; you may find yourself skipping stages or regressing to stages you already went through. The most productive stage, of course, is acceptance.

Denial: "This can't be *happening* to me!" If you are feeling disbelief or numbness about your diabetes, you might be in denial. A certain level of denial in the beginning can be positive because it protects you from over-worrying about all the possible outcomes of having a progressive disease.

Anger: "Why is this happening to *me*?" It's true that you didn't cause your own dia-betes; your genes played a big part. So it's not unnatural to be angry at having the condition. But anger is most useful when you channel it in a positive way—like becoming determined to do absolutely everything in your power to beat the disease.

Bargaining: If you're a person of faith you may catch yourself making deals with God, such as, "I'll be extra careful about eating healthy and exercising if you'll keep me off insulin." That's bargaining.

Depression: "I don't care anymore." This is the worst stage to get stuck in because when you're depressed you're much less likely to take good care of your health. If your depression lasts more than two weeks or becomes severe, call your doctor for help.

Acceptance: "I'm ready for whatever comes."

Focus on all the reasons that you'll succeed, not the reasons that you'll fail. You're eating better, you've started exercising more, your doctor recently put you on a new drug or changed the dosage, you're checking your blood sugar on schedule, and in general, you're a competent person who's succeeded at other things in life. In short, the deck is stacked in favor of you succeeding at managing your diabetes. Focus on these "success" cards in the deck, not on any perceived "doomed-to-fail" cards, like your weakness for bagels or past problems with your weight.

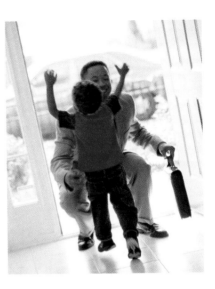

Keep a deity, a peace lily, or a worry stone on your desk. Choose a tangible object that symbolizes positive energy, tranquility, or victory to you, and keep it where you can see it during your day. Most times, it really doesn't take much to "check yourself back into" an attitude you can capitalize on and move forward with. Maybe your object is simply a shell from a beautiful beach or a trinket that's a sign of your faith. If you hit a rough patch in your day, hold, touch, or look at your object and think about what it means to you.

Post a picture of an inspirational person on your refrigerator or bathroom mirror. People who were successes despite huge obstacles are great reminders that "you can do it!" no matter what you face. Your hero might be Rosa Parks, Ghandi, or your own grandfather. You'll get an instant morale boost when you stop to comb your hair or make a meal and you see his or her face.

Don't say anything to yourself that you wouldn't say to someone else. Many of us are so used to being hard on ourselves that we don't even notice that we're doing it. What do you say to yourself when your blood sugar spikes or you forget to take a pill? Is it helpful or belittling? A good way to check is to ask, "Would I say this out loud to a friend?" If the answer is no, it's a good sign that you're not being fair to yourself or helpful to your cause. Instead, think of what you would say to a friend to be helpful and encouraging, and use that dialogue with yourself.

Pamper yourself at least once a month. Indulging in regular manicures, pedicures, massages, or haircuts will boost your self-esteem. Taking the time to give yourself some TLC reinforces the idea that you're worth it.

when diabetes gets you down

Having a glass-is-half-full outlook definitely helps people get through tough times—it's proven. But sometimes a long-term challenge like having diabetes just tires you out, leaving you feeling overwhelmed, frustrated, or plain old sad. What that happens, it's time to take action. Emotional and physical health are so closely intertwined that you really can't afford not to figure out what's getting you down and how to pull yourself back up again.

Talk to your diabetes educator. Unlike doctors, who have limited time to spend with you, certified diabetes educators (CDEs) have more time to answer questions and are there to help you solve frustrations. If you're feeling overwhelmed with your medication regimen or you don't understand why you're not seeing better results, don't keep it to yourself; diabetes is a big issue to tackle, and there's no reason to go it alone.

Join an online diabetes community. Sometimes there's nothing better than talking with someone who knows what you're going through. Through online discussion boards you can find people who share the very same challenges you're facing—and listen to how they solved them. You could create your own blog and post how you are doing each day, or take part in an existing one. Either way you'll have a place where you can go whenever you feel you need to soak up some support or to get out of your own head by helping others with your disease. The American Diabetes Association and the Joslin Diabetes Center both offer message boards for people with diabetes (www.diabetes.org and www.joslin.org).

Look for a stress management class at a nearby hospital. Chronic stress might be especially harmful to people with diabetes because it can raise blood sugar and shelve your motivation to eat healthy and exercise. Plus, depression, which is a common response to stress, raises the risk of heart disease. When Duke University researchers provided more than 100 people with diabetes-education classes—some with and some without stress-relief training—those who got the stress-relief training improved their blood sugar significantly compared to those who didn't.

Angry? Scared? Pretend that you are a caring friend, and write yourself a letter. You will have days when you just don't want to have diabetes. That's completely

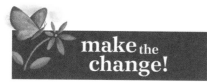

make the change!

The habit: Exercising whether you feel like it or not.

The benefit: A significantly improved mood.

The proof: Numerous studies make it crystal-clear that exercise improves depression if you do it regularly. In a study of more than 150 men and women aged 50 and over with major depression, regular aerobic exercise over the course of four months (30 minutes of moderately intense walking or jogging three times a week) was shown to be just as effective as antidepressant medications. A single exercise session can also boost your mood and help give you the energy to do it again.

normal. It's when you closet your worries, fears, and frustrations without addressing them that they eventually get bigger. It's great to be able to call a friend when you're feeling lousy, but if no one is around, be your own best friend. Grab a piece of paper, or sit down at your e-mail, and send yourself a message. What would you say to someone who was feeling like you are? Be kind, gentle, and supportive.

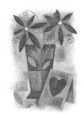

Lift your chest and roll your shoulders back and down for an instant boost. An uplifted posture can actually lead to an uplifted attitude, while slumping reinforces a defeated mindset.

You are not your disease, and having diabetes doesn't mean you're a failure.

Wear bright colors to improve your mood. It sounds trite, but it can really work. If you're used to wearing beige, gray, or black, pull out a shirt that's red or lime green, and wear it all day. Other people will perceive a more positive attitude in you, and their perceptions can actually "color" your real mood for the brighter!

Write down five things you like about yourself. Keep adding to your list regularly, whenever you think of a strength or positive quality. Include things you are good at doing, such as knitting, cooking, or being funny. If someone complements you, add it. On those days when you feel like your diabetes is getting the better of you, pull out your list—reviewing it will remind you that you are not your disease, and that having diabetes doesn't mean you're a failure.

Ask your spouse or a close friend what they love about you. Sometimes when you're feeling really lousy it can be hard to think of anything nice to say about yourself. That's when talking to someone you trust can really help. Consider writing down what your love or pal tells you, or ask them to send it an e-mail or letter that you can read whenever you need a boost.

Back out of one activity. If you're having a rough day and feeling overwhelmed, cut yourself some slack. If you have a mental to-do list, prioritize the items and move the bottom one to a day or two later. If your mother calls, tell her honestly that you don't have time to talk and will call her back tomorrow when you can spend more time with her on the phone.

Put your legs up on a wall to lower stress. Legs-up-the-wall is a favorite of yoga practitioners. They say that this pose not only relieves tired cramped feet and legs, it pulls the plug on stress. Place a pillow next to a wall and position yourself so your hips and low back are on the pillow, your head and shoulders are on the floor, and your legs are resting against the wall. Your body will be in the shape of an L. Close your eyes and breathe deeply for about a minute. If having your legs straight up a wall is uncomfortable, you can do the move by draping your legs up on a sofa or chair.

Write down your exact fears. Are you feeling scared that something terrible might happen as a consequence of your diabetes? Don't let a vague sense of anxiety eat away at you. Figure out—specifically—what you're afraid of and write it down in black and white so you can look at it objectively. Then ask yourself how likely this scenario really is and what concrete steps you can take to prevent it. Your certified diabetes educator can help you put your finger on both.

Can't figure out what's eating you? HALT! It's an oldie but goodie: Anytime something's eating at you—you're irritable, feeling sad, or can't shake a feeling of doom—stop and ask yourself if you are Hungry, Angry, Lonely, or Tired (HALT). If it's been too long since your last meal, you might be feeling irritable because your blood sugar is low. If it's anger you're feeling, you need to pinpoint what it is that has you upset, so you can work

The Diabetes–Depression Link

Having diabetes doesn't just try your emotional resources, it actually makes you more prone to depression. Scientists aren't sure why, but 20 percent of people with diabetes experience it. The link may be insulin resistance, which can raise the level of the stress hormone cortisol in the body—and high cortisol levels have been associated with depression. The happy news: Getting treatment for either depression or diabetes will help the other condition, too.

While everyone will have occasional days when they feel so wiped out that they won't have the energy to make a healthy salad for lunch or get out and walk, you should know when your symptoms mean something more serious. If you've been experiencing five or more of the following signs and symptoms for two weeks or longer, you could be clinically depressed and should see a doctor or qualified mental health professional for evaluation and help.

• You feel persistently sad or anxious.
• Your sleep patterns have changed (wanting to sleep all the time or not being able to fall or stay asleep).
• You're experiencing a loss of appetite and weight loss, or an increase in appetite and weight gain.
• You have lost your pleasure and interest in previously enjoyable activities.
• You are frequently restless or irritable.
• You have difficulty concentrating, remembering, or making decisions.
• You feel constantly fatigued or drained of energy.
• You constantly feel guilty, hopeless, or worthless.
• You are thinking about suicide or death.

through it. Lonely? Call a friend. Finally, have you been getting enough sleep? Being overly fatigued can throw off your mood.

Buy lemon- or orange-scented potpourri. The refreshing aroma of citrus has been found in studies to boost mood and reduce anxiety. You can find aromatherapy oils in health food stores, or look for citrus-scented potpour-ri, candles, or incense sticks in gift stores. Keep several small bowls around your house. Even simpler: cut half an orange, eat the fruit, then squeeze the rind into the air.

Plant an herb garden. Rosemary and peppermint are two plants that have been shown to perk you up, with a nice bonus of dampening appetite. Lavender is known to have a calming effect. Plant these herbs in your yard and take cuttings to keep in a small glass of water in your kitchen. You'll get a nice whiff every time you go near your fridge.

Slowly blow out an imaginary candle when you feel stressed. Deep breathing elicits a relaxation response in your body. Unfortunately, most of us take short, shallow breaths—especially when we're feeling anxious—that add to our stress levels by robbing the body of needed oxygen. Counteract this tendency by pretending that there's a candle about three feet in front of you. Take a slow deep breath in, then exhale slowly and completely to blow it out. Repeat three to five times.

Look at something green at least once a day. Nature's a proven stress reliever and mood booster, and there's no need to go farther than your own backyard to get the benefits. Pick up and examine a pretty leaf or flower, or watch a little sparrow hopping about. Most of us spend our days focus-ing on tasks. Taking a time out to contemplate something completely different gives your mind a chance to relax and refresh.

Have weekly laugh-it-up dates. Getting together with a rowdy group of friends, making a date to go see a comedian with your spouse, or just taking yourself out to a comedy or renting a funny movie can perk you up when you are feeling down. Bonus: Laughing boosts your heart health, according to a study from the University of Maryland Medical Center in Baltimore. Researchers there found that of 300 adults, those who had heart disease were 40 percent less likely to laugh than those without heart troubles.

Blow your stack? Have a get-out-of-jail free card handy. Remember these cards in your old Monopoly game? You can either rifle through your game closet and pull out one of the real cards or get an index card and write "Get out of jail free." Below that, add, "This card may be used to remind me that I'm only human and humans make mistakes—I'm now off the hook!"

overcoming obstacles

Ever watch a hurdler on the track field? They propel their bodies over those hurdles as if they weren't even there. Sooner or later, you're bound to run into your own hurdles when it comes to taking good care of your diabetes. They simply come with the territory. The trick is to set yourself up to fly over them so you don't end up face-down on the track.

Get enough sleep. Anyone who's sleep-deprived copes badly with challenges. If you're well rested, you'll be more resilient and better able to face the issues that come your way with an "I can handle this" attitude.

Sign up for a diabetes class. Look for one on the specific issue you're having trouble with, such as using an insulin pump, or go to a general diabetes class if that's all that's available and ask your questions there.

Join a weekly or monthly diabetes support group. Remember, you are far from alone in this battle. There are 180 million people worldwide who have diabetes. Take advantage of it. Studies show that people who have

Getting to the Bottom of Diabetes Burnout

Many people newly diagnosed with diabetes start out motivated to make all the necessary changes to take care of themselves. But as time goes by, it's common to start feeling drained or overwhelmed, something experts refer to as "diabetes burnout." Figuring out your level of burnout is key to relighting your fire, says William Polonsky, PhD, CDE, diabetes psychologist and author of *Diabetes Burnout.*

How Burned Out Are You?

Ask yourself if the six statements below are true or false.

1. My diabetes is taking up too much of my mental and physical energy every day.

2. I feel too exhausted, fatigued, or "burned out" by the constant effort it takes to manage my diabetes.

3. I feel like I am often failing with my diabetes regimen.

4. I feel like diabetes controls my life.

5. I'm not motivated to keep up with my diabetes treatment plan.

6. I feel completely overwhelmed about my diabetes.

If you answered true to more than two of the above, you may be experiencing burnout. Your first step is to talk to your doctor, a certified diabetes educator, or a counselor. Maybe your medications or shots can be adjusted so that you don't have to take so many throughout your day. Or maybe counseling will help you learn new strategies for easing stress and improving your mood.

golden rule!   Confront Your Fears About Insulin Before You Need It

More than half of people with type 2 diabetes will eventually need insulin if they live with the disease long enough. Having a conversation with your doctor *before* he needs to pull out the big gun can help allay your fears. The fact is, it isn't really the insulin or the needles that scare most people; it's what they stand for—a worsening of this progressive disease. If your doctor does suggest insulin, it's probably because your blood sugars are too high. Insulin helps you regain control and can improve your health, and the way you feel, immensely. And keeping your blood sugar under better control will slash your risk of serious diabetes-related complications. Discuss your fears with your doctor at your next appointment, and find out what his guidelines are for when he will suggest insulin.

support are more resistant to the damage of stress than those who go it alone. Ask your doctor, check at your local hospital, or search online at www.diabetes.org for a local support group. You'll find plenty of people who've faced similar obstacles and found solutions.

Work with your doctor. Don't be afraid to troubleshoot with your doctor about problems you're having. Do you feel like your diabetes medication is causing you to gain weight? Weight gain is indeed a side effect of some diabetes drugs. Your doctor might be able to switch you to another.

Role-play difficult situations. If you dread being asked about why you won't eat cake or drink alcohol, you feel like you can't ask the doctor the questions you want answered, or you have an overbearing family member you don't know how to confront, practice how you'll handle the situation next time with a close friend or a counselor playing the other part. This way you can fine-tune your approach before you have to use it.

Empower yourself with information. Ignorance is not bliss, especially for people with diabetes. When your blood sugar fluctuates wildly, or you get dizzy for no apparent reason, it can be scary. Talk to your doctor or certified diabetes educator about what could be causing the problem and what you can do to fix it. Remember, knowledge is power.

Too many doughnuts in your day? Work with a registered dietitian. Sticking to a healthy eating plan can be a major bugaboo for many people. If you are struggling with food, ask your doctor for a referral to a registered dietitian. This expert will analyze how you are eating, help you pinpoint your pitfalls, and offer suggestions for healthier meals and strategies for overcoming temptations.

keep your motivation stoked

Having diabetes requires daily attention: checking your blood sugar, taking your medications, watching your diet, getting exercise. All of this requires a motivated frame of mind. The real challenge is maintaining that enthusiasm to take good care of yourself over the long haul. Use these inspirational strategies and incentives to keep you going.

Give yourself a gold star whenever you achieve even the smallest success. If you made it out the door for a walk (even if it was just 10 minutes), if you lost one pound, or your blood sugar numbers were a little steadier this week, take notice and give yourself some recognition! Buy a sheet of gold star stickers from an office supply store and put them in your blood sugar log, your food log, or your exercise log—wherever one belongs. Success breeds more success, especially when you feel like you're on a roll.

Don't cancel that doctor's appointment! Staying on top of your medical care will lower your risk of complications, injuries, and illness. This includes regular doctor's visits, but also regular visits to the dentist, foot doctor, and eye doctor.

If you're trying to lose weight, keep a food diary. People with diabetes who are trying to shed extra pounds are more successful if they keep a written record of their daily food intake.

Check in with supportive friends once a week. Having cheerleaders to share even little successes with, such as avoiding French fries for a week or going walking for 10 minutes on an extra-busy day, can help you feel empowered and capable. Create a group of e-mail buddies, or have one or two friends you can call at least once a week.

Signs of Success

When you have diabetes, signs that you're managing it well go beyond your blood sugar numbers. Include any of these in your mental "success log."

• Lower blood sugar peaks
• Fewer episodes of hypoglycemia
• Improved cholesterol levels

• Lower blood pressure
• More energy
• Better-fitting clothes
• A smaller waistline
• Improved moods
• Better sleep
• Greater stamina
• Higher self-esteem

golden rule! Remember What's at Stake

According to the American Association of Clinical Endocrinologists, an estimated three out of five Americans with diabetes have one or more complications associated with the disease. The way to avoid them is to keep your blood sugar in line by taking your medication or insulin and following the lifestyle tips in this book. The good news: The United Kingdom Prospective Diabetes Study, a 10-year study of over 5,000 patients with newly diagnosed type 2 diabetes, found that eye damage, kidney damage, and nerve damage were reduced significantly in study subjects who kept their blood sugar under tight control (a median A1C of 7 percent). The study also found that aggressive control of high blood pressure significantly reduced cardiovascular complications and retinopathy in people with type 2 diabetes.

Keep a daily diary. You don't have to be Anne Frank or Anaïs Nin, writing page after page of deep meaningful feelings. Just doing a quick check-in on paper can keep you centered and focused on your goals. Include how you felt for most of the day and note any highs or lows (physically or emotionally). Plus, if you write regularly, then the days when your thoughts do runneth over, you'll know where to put them.

Develop a personal mantra. Repeat it to yourself any time you're feeling grumpy, stressed, or bummed out. The phrase can be as simple as "Life happens" or "Don't sweat the small stuff." If you can't think of anything, search for inspirational quotes on the Web. If you're a worrier, maybe you should remember the Swedish proverb: "Worry often gives a small thing a big shadow." If you're feeling blue, maybe the Confucius saying, "Our greatest glory is not in never falling, but in rising every time we fall," will speak to you. And there's no one better at pure inspiration than Ghandi, who said, "My life is my message."

Do a crossword, Sudoku, or jigsaw puzzle. When your efforts to bring down your blood sugar or lose weight just aren't showing results (yet), it can really leave you feeling frustrated. Sometimes the best thing to do is to forget all about your diabetes for a short time and distract yourself with a simple crossword puzzle or other game or activity that has a finishing point. You'll get a break from what's bothering you and have a reminder that there are some things within your control.

Watch a comedy or nature show, not a tearjerker. If you've been having trouble with dishes of candy at work or too much pasta on spaghetti night, avoid the four-hankie show at the cinema. An Australian study found that women who watched a sad documentary were much more

whip it together! Double-Rich Chocolate Pudding Treat

When you want a little reward for a week's worth of very healthy eating, look to this rich, creamy treat. Remember, nutritionists say it's good to enjoy your favorite foods once in a while, in moderation, so you don't end up feeling deprived.

In a heavy saucepan, combine ⅓ cup **Splenda**, 3 tablespoons **flour**, and 3 tablespoons **cocoa powder**. Stir in 2¼ cups **fat-free milk** and cook over medium heat until thickened and bubbly. Cook and stir for 1 more minute. Remove from the heat. Stir in 1 ounce grated **bittersweet chocolate**, 2 teaspoons **butter**, and 1½ teaspoon **vanilla**. Spoon into dishes and cover with plastic wrap.

likely to overindulge on chocolates than a group that watched a gorgeous travel movie. Another study from the University of Mississippi found that people munched nearly 30 percent more buttered popcorn when they watched "Love Story" compared to when they saw the comedy "Sweet Home Alabama."

Schedule 15 minutes per day to do absolutely nothing. Write it in your planner or schedule a repeating break on your computer calendar. Whether you use the time to just sit quietly, to take an easy stroll, or to repeat a positive phrase to yourself, having a few minutes of "off-the-clock" time refreshes your mind and helps you let go of stress or worrywart thinking. Taking small breaks from your tasks can even give you more energy to attack them.

Take a class for pure fun. Be it a yoga, painting, pottery, cooking, or belly-dancing class, it can help you avoid feeling like your whole life is about your diabetes. You'll also tap into your creative side, which is always a sure-fire way to feel more energized and upbeat.

Connect with a place of worship every weekend. Staying close to your faith on a regular basis can help you socially and emotionally. You'll have the opportunity to connect to others who share your beliefs, as well as time to be contemplative about your purpose in life. If religion isn't for you, a meditation or other support group might offer the same sort of community.

Do a good deed at least once a day. Take the time to hold a door open for someone who's carrying loads of bags, carry flowers to a neighbor who is homebound, or give someone a compliment. Doing something nice for someone else is a great way to get out of your own head when you are feeling lousy. It also makes you feel good.

chapter fifteen

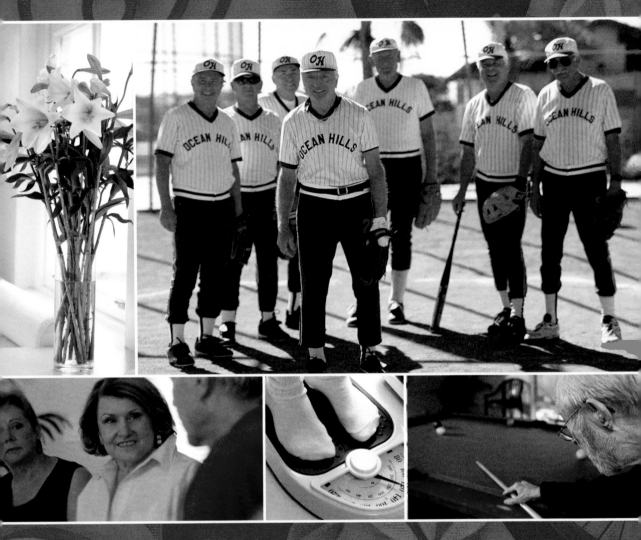

in your life

Life happens, as the saying goes. Everyone gets sick now and then and has bugaboos to deal with, from gaining weight to smoking. Read on to discover ways to keep *your* life on a healthy track.

find your focus

You block out time for your doctor's appointments and take the time to check your blood sugar levels regularly. Hopefully you also make time to cook and eat healthy meals and to get some exercise at least several days a week. But you need "you time" on a regular basis, too—time for peace, relaxation, and quiet contemplation. It's also important to nurture your soul to keep stress and depression—two significant enemies of people with diabetes—at bay.

Go "on strike" from your life for a week. Do you have too much on your to-do list, and not enough time in which to do it? Let everything go—the errands, laundry, house cleaning, and whatever else is causing you stress—for the next seven days. When you find that life goes on even if you don't pick up your dry cleaning or dust your vertical blinds, you'll have a new perspective on whether it's worth it to drive yourself crazy trying to get it all done. Maybe one or two undone chores really did create a kink in your life—say, not going to the grocery store. Now you know what should be at the top of your list the next time!

Carve your exercise in stone. When life starts to burst at the seams, it may be tempting to let your exercise plans slide. Don't do anything of the sort; let something else slide instead. In the end, exercise actually boosts your energy level. It also helps melt away stress. In one study published in the *Journal of the American Medical Association,* getting aerobic exercise for 35 minutes three times a week had the same beneficial effects on stress and depression as attending stress management classes for 90 minutes each week. Exercise is also an excellent outlet for your frustrations.

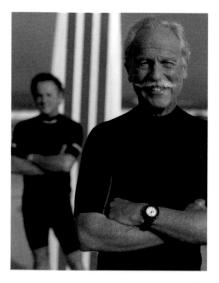

Women: Schedule some indulgences. Taking care of your family and taking care of your diabetes are both huge responsibilities, and it's not hard to feel like you've been lost in the shuffle. Make a conscious effort to take care of good old you, too. (Remember, your life wouldn't run very well without you in it.) Formally write at least one self-indulgence on your calendar every week. Treat these pleasures as the important appointments that they are, and stick to the schedule. You might plan lunch with a dear friend, a manicure, a movie by yourself, or a whole Saturday morning working in your garden.

Take up a hobby in which you get moving *and* meet people. Few things are more energizing than meeting a new friend, especially at a certain age. But it may take

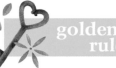

golden rule!   Nudge Your Friends Away from Restaurants

If you and your friends are stuck in the rut of meeting for meals out, it's time to shake things up. Seek out opportunities to spend time together that have more to do with fun and activity than with food. Decide as a group to join a bowling league or learn to play bocce ball, or get together at someone's house to knit and gossip. Become the "what's happening" expert of your group by scouring the entertainment listings of your newspaper, checking community Web sites, and checking the calendars at the YMCA and other community centers.

---

a bold move on your part to get out there and do it. If you've always wanted to try rock climbing, go for it, even if you think you're over the hill. You never know who you might meet at the climbing wall (and keep in mind that it's good to have a few friends who are younger than you), and their encouragement could be priceless. Or make model airplanes and fly them at a local club, learn horseback riding, or join a group that reenacts historic battles—you'll likely make friends from all walks of life, and stoke a passion that reminds you why you want to stick around on this Earth for as long as possible.

If you're feeling overwhelmed, see a counselor. Some of the happiest, most successful people you can name have used a therapist, counselor, or psychologist to get them through stressful times. Ask your doctor or certified diabetes educator about finding a counselor who has experience in dealing with issues related to diabetes—they get inquiries like that all of the time. Or approach your clergy if you belong to a church.

Become a regular at your house of worship. Researchers say that practicing your faith regularly can pay off not just emotionally but also physically. One survey found that people who did not attend church every week had a 21 percent greater chance of dying from circulatory diseases (which diabetes patients are particularly vulnerable to) than people who did. A study of stroke survivors revealed that the more religious the patient was, the less likely he was to have anxiety or depression, both of which can hinder recuperation. Researchers suspect that people who attend a place of worship regularly benefit from a stronger social network and receive more encouragement than people who don't regularly attend.

Keep your closest pals on speed dial. It sounds odd to say that having close friends is an important factor in controlling your diabetes, but it's true in several ways. Having people around you who care about you could make the difference between your sticking to your disease management efforts and letting them slide. Friends who care about you are encouraging workout partners and will keep in mind your dietary needs when they invite you over for dinner. When you have a strong emotional support system, you have a greater sense of identity—within a community and as an individual—which helps you weather whatever emotional difficulties life throws your way.

Lend a hand to those who need one. There are hundreds of people in your community who need you, and helping them could help you in ways you'd never imagine. The most important thing you'll glean from volunteering is perspective—that having diabetes, in the grand scope of things, is not as big a burden to bear as what some others have to endure. Volunteering at a soup kitchen or coaching a youth basketball group at a homeless shelter will not only lend perspective, it may get you moving around more!

Adopt a pet. Pet ownership is known to lower blood pressure, reduce stress, and make people feel less lonely. Exactly how people benefit from their relationships with pets is not fully understood, but scientists suspect that this bond fulfills a human need to be close to other living beings. In a German survey of 10,000 people, the people who owned pets required 10 percent fewer doctor visits over a five-year period than people who didn't. A survey in the United States showed that heart attack victims were twice as likely to survive for a year when they had a pet at home.

The Power of Prayer

Want to live seven years longer? Start praying. We're not joking here; seven years is the increase in lifespan you can expect if you nurture your soul and your health through prayer, faith, and religious involvement, according to various studies. For one thing, research shows a strong connection between heart health and religious faith. In one study, people who went into open-heart surgery and reported feeling strength and comfort from their religion were three times more likely to survive the surgery than people with no such spiritual grounding. If there's a placebo effect at work here—if people get better because they believe they will—who's to argue with the benefits? Whether praying calms you, gives you hope, or helps you tend to your inner self, if you feel you're getting something out of it, it's time well spent.

prepare for sick days

You wake up with a fever, a stuffy nose, or a sore throat. Your first instinct may be to call your boss and say you'll be out sick or to cancel other plans you had for the day. Your second instinct should be to take care of yourself *and* your diabetes, since being sick can throw your blood sugar out of whack. It's important to have a plan in place before you get sick, not when your head is all fuzzy. Here's a general game plan; ask your doctor if there is other advice he wants you to follow.

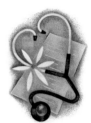

Being sick can spike your blood sugar, so check your levels more often.

Know when to call your doctor. It's a good idea to inform your doctor if you get sick, especially if you are unable to eat, have diarrhea, or have been vomiting for more than six hours. You should also make the call if you have had a fever that is not improving, cracked lips, or flushed skin for longer than two days.

Continue all your medications. Some people make the mistake of skipping medications or insulin when they are so sick that they don't feel like eating, but it is especially important to keep taking all prescription drugs, especially because being sick can raise your blood sugar. If you take insulin, your doctor may even suggest that you adjust (usually increase) the dosage when you are down for the count.

Check your blood sugar more frequently. When you start to get sick, your body goes on the defensive, sending out hormones to fight the illness. This is good news, of course, but the battle your body wages can spike your blood sugar and reduce your ability to use insulin. Usually your doctor will recommend that you check your blood sugar every three to four hours when you are feeling poorly, but be sure to discuss specific recommendations with her before you get sick. If your blood sugar readings are high when you are sick (exact levels should be discussed with your doctor), she may recommend extra insulin.

Ask your doctor about checking your ketones. When you're sick, if your blood sugar levels are consistently above 240 mg/dl, you'll want to do a urine ketone test (available in drugstores) to check for diabetes ketoacidosis, in which the body resorts to breaking down fat for energy and releases ketones, which poison the blood. Though it's rare in people with type 2 diabetes, the condition can lead to coma and even death. Signs of ketoacidosis are nausea, extreme thirst or dry mouth, stomach pain, vomiting, blurred vision, flushed skin or fever, trouble breathing or paying attention, weakness or drowsiness, loss of appetite, and a fruitlike breath odor. If your ketone levels are high, call your doctor immediately or go to the emergency room.

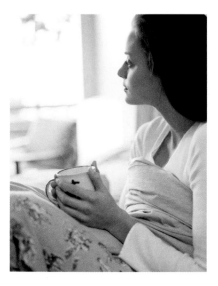

Keep "sick day" foods in the pantry. You may not have much of an appetite when you are sick, but it is important to eat as regularly as possible to help your blood sugar stay level. Try to choose foods from your regular healthy diet that are easy on the stomach such as oatmeal, chicken noodle soup, rice, applesauce, and toast. Stock your pantry with cans of broth-based soups, saltine-type crackers, regular gelatin, brown rice, and canned chicken broth, and fill your freezer with sorbet or fruit juice bars.

Consume at least a cup of fluid every hour. When your blood sugar is high, your body tries to flush glucose out of your system by making you urinate more. This puts you at risk for dehydration; that's why ramping up your fluid intake is crucial if you're not feeling well. If you can't keep food down, make up for that calorie loss by drinking sugary, caffeine-free fluids such as fruit juice, sports drinks, and non-diet soft drinks. Call your doctor if you're showing symptoms of dehydration, including dry mouth, dry skin, cracked lips, extreme thirst, mental confusion, and sunken eyes.

Get plenty of bed rest. It's true that physical activity will lower your blood sugar, but it isn't safe to exercise when you are sick. It's more important to rest to allow your immune system to work on making you better. If you are restless, dim the light in your room by pulling the shades, ask your spouse or friend to rent a DVD for you, or listen to some relaxing music.

***Before* you get sick, arrange for backup help.** When you're flat on your back nursing the flu and trying to manage your diabetes, you probably won't have much energy left to run your household. Before you are sidelined by illness, put plans in place to get the help you need. If you have kids, call a relative or the parents of your kids' closest friends and ask if they'd be willing to watch your kids on sick days (offer to reciprocate where appropriate). Get your spouse to commit to taking over chores when you're feeling ill, and let him fret about dirty dishes or stinky cat boxes.

tried-and-true paths to effective weight loss

Most people with type 2 diabetes struggle with their weight. And chances are, your doctor has given you little or no guidance on how to shed those extra pounds. But doing it will likely make your blood sugar easier to control and can lower your blood pressure and cholesterol, too. In many cases, doctors will allow patients who lose a significant amount of weight to cut back on—or eliminate—some of their medications. The best way to lighten your load? Steer clear of the hype and stick to proven strategies.

Set moderate, achievable weight-loss goals. Research from Indiana University in Indianapolis shows that most people think they have to drop 50 to 100 pounds to be "successful" at weight loss—a belief that sets them up for failure. Instead, start with a reasonable goal, like losing 10 pounds. Doctors say that kind of moderate weight loss still has a beneficial effect on diabetes—and if you reach that goal, you'll have the drive to lose 10 more pounds!

Know your Body Mass Index (BMI). To find out whether your body weight falls within the range of normal, overweight, or obese, consult a BMI table or an online BMI calculator. If you're good with numbers, whip out a pencil and paper and run through the formula presented on page 254 (see Calculating Your Body Mass Index). If your BMI is less than 25, your weight is normal. If your BMI is at least 25 but less than 30, you're overweight. If your BMI is 30 or above, you're considered obese.

Find a weight-loss buddy. Dieting with a buddy provides more than support—it can help you lose more weight. That's what a recent Brown University study of 109 people and their dieting partners found. Those with a motivated pal lost nearly twice as much weight as those who dieted solo. Having someone within walking distance can be an added bonus. Find three neighbors and announce your weight-loss intentions. Chances are they'll have some weight to lose as well.

Join a weight-loss group. When researchers at Columbia University in New York assigned 413 overweight and obese men and women to either a self-help program in which they met twice with a nutritionist

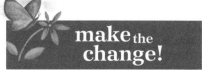

make the **change!**

The habit: Losing 10 to 15 pounds.

The result: Improving your chances of preventing diabetes or diabetes-related complications.

The proof: In a major American research study called the Diabetes Prevention Program, people with prediabetes were given instructions to lose 7 percent of their body weight (for a 150-pound person, that's 10.5 pounds) through diet and exercise and to keep the weight off for the duration of the three-year study. Their risk of developing type 2 diabetes dropped by 58 percent. The lifestyle changes worked particularly well for people age 60 and older, reducing their risk by 71 percent. If you already have diabetes, dropping 5 to 7 percent of your body weight can improve your insulin sensitivity, which in turn lowers blood sugar. It can also lower your cholesterol and blood pressure.

and then followed a program on their own or Weight Watchers, after two years those going to Weight Watchers lost more than those going it alone. You don't have to join Weight Watchers or other commercial weight-loss programs; you can also check local community centers, churches, or hospitals for weight-control programs or support groups.

Pair calorie-cutting with exercise. People who exercise as well as cut calories have an easier time losing weight and keeping it off than people who just cut calories. Burning an extra 250 calories a day—about the amount used in a brisk 45-minute walk—lops off about 26 pounds a year, as long as you don't replace those calories with food.

Eat breakfast. Fiber helps you stay full, and a good way to get a healthy dose is to eat a breakfast cereal that contains at least 5 grams of fiber per serving. Breakfast does more than provide fiber, though. Studies show that eating breakfast helps you eat less food later in the day—and consume fewer total calories.

Aim to lose weight *slowly*. You can shave off just one pound a week—or even two pounds a month—by making small adjustments in your eating and physical activity. Don't let fad diet advertisements dazzle you with "miracle" plans in which you can lose 100 pounds in two months. Researchers say that people who achieve weight loss in such programs typically gain back most or all of the weight within five years. You're far better off to learn how to make the lifestyle changes that will keep the weight off permanently, even if it means slower weight loss. What's more, crash diets that deprive you of essential nutrients can be very dangerous. If you need guidance, enlist the assistance of your doctor, registered dietitian, or a reputable weight loss program such as Weight Watchers.

Ask a registered dietitian to design an eating plan for you. It may not even seem like a weight-loss plan if she integrates your favorite foods! A registered dietitian is trained to help you set reasonable calorie goals and

Calculating Your Body Mass Index

To calculate your BMI, multiply your weight in pounds by 703. Divide the answer by your height in inches. Then divide that answer by your height in inches.

If you weigh 150 pounds and you're 65 inches tall, you have a BMI of 24.96 (150 x 703 = 105450 / 65 / 65 = 24.96).

whip it together! Breakfast Parfait

Starting your morning out right with a really delicious and healthy breakfast can keep you on the track of eating well all day long. This sweet and crunchy parfait does the trick.

Add ½ teaspoon **sugar substitute** and 2 teaspoons **orange juice** to ½ cup **blueberries**. Let stand for 15 minutes. In a tall glass, make a layer of ¼ cup nonfat **Greek yogurt** (if unavailable, use regular plain yogurt and pour off excess water), ½ teaspoon lightly ground **flaxseeds**, and ¼ of the blueberries. Repeat the layers until all ingredients are used.

make sure that you're getting the vitamins and minerals you need to help you manage your diabetes.

Keep a food diary for five days. Log *everything* you eat and drink, even if it's just water, a bite of ice cream, or a breath mint. Your entries should include the time of day, size and number of servings, calories (a calorie-counting paperback book will help), what emotions you were feeling at the time, or any other circumstances that happened just before you ate. Food diaries are eye-openers for many people because so many of us eat without thinking about it. Review your food diary with your registered dietitian; she'll help you identify situations or emotions that may cause you to overeat. These diaries can also be great tools for managing diabetes because they'll help you remember what you ate that sent your blood sugar soaring, and what keeps you on an even keel.

Supplement with calcium. Losing weight can trigger bone loss, so if you're a woman, make sure you're supplementing with 500 to 600 milligrams of calcium twice a day. Choose a calcium supplement that also contains vitamin D.

Consider bariatric surgery as a last resort. So-called "stomach-stapling" surgery can have dramatically positive effects on some people's diabetes, practically reversing the condition. But don't take gastric bypass lightly; it's major surgery, so it's not without risks, including a 1 percent risk of death from the surgery itself. Weight-loss surgery is recommended only for people who are severely obese (usually with a body mass index of 40 or more, but if you have diabetes, 35 or more) and can't lose weight any other way. Those who have surgery have to commit to serious lifestyle changes: They will only be able to eat small meals, may need dietary supplements and perhaps medications, and will require frequent medical checkups. The cost of this surgery is substantial, too, and some insurance companies won't cover it.

stamp out your cigarette addiction

Here's an ugly statistic: Some 90 percent of people with diabetes who have a foot amputated are smokers. If you're a smoker with diabetes, quitting should be your top priority. Diabetes is already putting your heart and blood vessels at risk, and the last thing you need is added damage from cigarettes. Smoking narrows your blood vessels, which can damage your heart; in some cases, it can lead to impotence and foot amputation. As someone with diabetes, you're already at high risk of developing kidney disease, nerve damage, and eye damage; smoking increases your chances of developing all three.

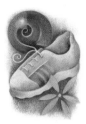

Smokers who exercise are twice as likely to quit.

Decide why want you want to quit. About 70 percent of people who smoke say they want to quit. But tobacco's addictive, there's no two ways about it. So for most people, quitting isn't easy. If better health isn't motivation enough, think about quitting for the sake of your loved ones. Whom will you miss, or who will miss you most, if you die more than a decade prematurely? Quit for them.

Stick motivational photos on the fridge. Want to be around for your granddaughter's wedding in 20 years? Put her smiling face on your fridge. Looking forward to retiring with your spouse and driving an RV cross-country? Grab a magazine and cut out a picture of an RV like the one you want, post it, and imagine yourself in it every day.

Zero in on when and why you smoke. Keep a list of the times of day and situations in which you're most likely to light up. Understanding when you most "need" a cigarette will help you devise things to do instead of smoking. If you need to have something to do with your hands while talking on the phone, fiddle with a pen or a small paperweight. If you like a cigarette with your morning coffee, start drinking tea instead. If a smoking break at work gives you an energy boost, instead go for a brisk walk around the parking lot.

Exercise regularly. It can help you quit smoking by burning off stress hormones so you feel less of an urge to smoke and by producing feel-good brain chemicals to help reduce the uncomfortable effects of nicotine withdrawal. A Gallup Poll found that smokers who exercised were twice as likely to quit as their sedentary counterparts. Daily exercise can also help you avoid the dreaded five- to 10-pound weight gain commonly associated with kicking the habit.

Tell everyone you know that you're quitting. When your family, friends, and coworkers all know you are trying to give up cigarettes, they'll give you encouragement and will be less likely to put you in tempting situations. And when you know that you're accountable to everyone around you, you will be less likely to sneak away for a puff.

Give yourself a smoke-free deadline. Pick a date in the near future when you won't have any major stress to deal with. If your daughter is getting married in three weeks, or if you're moving, changing jobs, or hosting a house full of relatives soon, push off your quit date until after the chaos has died down. The more stressed out you are, the stronger your cravings (and withdrawal symptoms) will likely be.

Choose the cessation method that will work best for you. If you're a casual smoker, you may be able to just quit cold turkey. But if you're a heavy smoker, you may need to wean yourself off nicotine by means of nicotine patches or chewing gum or by using nasal sprays or inhalers. (Some of these treatments are available over-the-counter, and some are available by prescription.) If you're comfortable with alternative treatments, hypnosis and acupuncture may also help.

If you use the patch, keep a watchful eye on your blood sugar. Nicotine patches can raise glucose levels; you'll want to check your blood sugar more frequently than you typically do so that you get a good sense of how the patch affects you. And never smoke while you're on nicotine patches— nicotine can be toxic in large doses, and the combination of patch and tobacco could be deadly.

Ask your doctor if stop-smoking prescriptions might be right for you. There are a couple of prescription medications on the market that may help you kick the habit. Varenicline will reduce the kick you get from nicotine while alleviating withdrawal symptoms. Buproprion will reduce cravings for nicotine; it will even relieve symptoms of depression for some people.

Trash your smoking paraphernalia. When you don't have ashtrays, lighters, cigarettes, or other tobacco-related accessories in your home, it will be all the more difficult for you to light up on impulse.

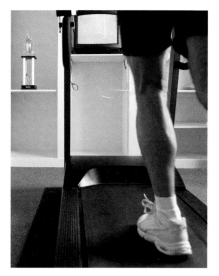

Have your curtains, clothes, and rugs professionally laundered. Do whatever it takes to banish the stale-smoke scent that your home might have. Smoke permeates just about every kind of fabric; if you smoke indoors, chances are your home smells stale, and you're so used to it that you don't even notice the odor. Once all of your appointments have been professionally laundered, you'll see how fresh "smoke-free" living can smell.

And remembering all the money you just spent to get everything clean may just keep you from pulling out another cigarette.

Make your home a no-smoking zone. Post "no smoking" signs, banish ashtrays, and make clear to visitors that they shouldn't light up under your roof. It's your house—if you have made the commitment not to smoke, no one else should be allowed to smoke under your watch, either!

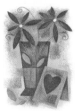

Don't give up. Most people have to try to quit several times.

Create diversions. Smoking is a pastime as much as an addiction. You smoke for something to do during breaks at work, while driving your car, and during quiet evenings at home. Once you quit, you'll feel that something is missing during these times. Fill the space with other activity. Sip water and sing along to a favorite CD while you drive. Take short walks instead of coffee breaks. Choose hands-on activities such as crocheting or refinishing furniture to do as you wind down in the evening. You'll miss cigarettes less if you keep busy.

Take 10. When the urge to light up strikes, look at your watch and give yourself 10 minutes. During that time, take full, deep breaths as you would if you were drawing on a cigarette. Deep breathing will fill your lungs with clean, smoke-free air and trigger a relaxation response. By the time 10 minutes is up, the acute urge to smoke will have passed, and you'll be better able to move past the craving.

Take a stop-smoking class. This may be just the ticket if you need group support in banishing tobacco from your life. Often employers, health insurance companies, and hospitals offer such classes. You can also ask your doctor for a referral, or check with cancer, heart health, or lung health associations.

If you relapse with smoking, quit again … and again. Don't give up! Most people have to try to kick the habit several times before they're finally successful. Your first three smoke-free months will be the hardest. While you are battling cravings, remind yourself that doing without tobacco won't always be this uncomfortable or difficult. In the meantime, avoid alcohol, which will lower your resolve, and avoid other people who are smoking.

Get away from second-hand smoke, too. Hanging out with smokers not only tempts fate, it also hurts your heart. Persistent exposure to cigarette smoke, either at home or on the job, nearly doubles your risk of having a heart attack even if you don't smoke, according to a landmark 10-year study of more than 32,000 women. If you socialize with smokers, do so in nonsmoking establishments, where they can puff outdoors. If you live with a smoker, take the ashtray outside and keep it there.

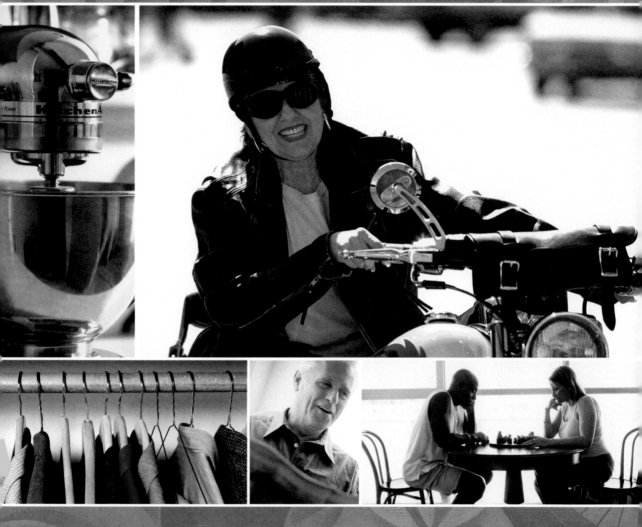

tools

Staying on top of your diabetes means staying on top
of your meals, your medication, your blood sugar levels, your
doctor visits, and more. Use these handy tools and charts to make
living healthy a little easier.

diabetes testing
and management schedule

At Every Doctor's Visit (usually 4 times per year)

Test	Date	Result	Date	Result	Date	Result	Date	Result
A1C (goal is lower than 7)								
Blood pressure (goal is lower than 130/80)								
Foot check		///		///		///		///

Twice a Year

Test	Date	Date
Dental cleaning and exam		

Yearly (on anniversary of last test)

Test	Last Year's Date	Last Year's Result	This Year's Date	This Year's Result
Microalbumin urine test (for kidney function)		///		///
Eye exam (with dilation)		///		///
LDL cholesterol*				
HDL cholesterol**				
Triglycerides***				
Foot exam (from a podiatrist)		///		///
Flu shot		///		///

*goal is lower than 100 mg/dl or lower than 70 mg/dl if you have known cardiovascular disease

**goal is higher than 40 mg/dl for men and higher than 50 mg/dl for women

***goal is lower than 150 mg/dl

planning for your next doctor's visit

Date and time of appointment: _____

Name of doctor: _____

Name of certified diabetes educator: _____

Name of registered dietitian: _____

I need to bring the following to my appointment:

❑ A list of my medications
❑ My glucose meter
❑ My glucose log book
❑ A record of any test or examination I had other than in my doctor's office
❑ My food diary
❑ My physical activity log
❑ Other: _____
_____

Check if any tests need to be done prior to appointment:

❑ A1C
❑ Urine test of protein to check kidney function
❑ Dilated eye exam
❑ Cholesterol and triglycerides
❑ Other: _____
_____

Questions to ask:

1. _____
_____
_____

2. _____
_____
_____

3. _____
_____
_____

4. _____
_____
_____

medication record

Name: _____

What it's for: _____

Amount: _____ How often: _____

When to take: _____

Name: _____

What it's for: _____

Amount: _____ How often: _____

When to take: _____

Name: _____

What it's for: _____

Amount: _____ How often: _____

When to take: _____

Name: _____

What it's for: _____

Amount: _____ How often: _____

When to take: _____

Name: _____

What it's for: _____

Amount: _____ How often: _____

When to take: _____

Name: _____

What it's for: _____

Amount: _____ How often: _____

When to take: _____

Name: _____

What it's for: _____

Amount: _____ How often: _____

When to take: _____

weekly blood sugar log

Use this chart to log the results of your blood sugar checks for an overall snapshot of your blood sugar control over the course of a day and a week. Bring these log sheets to your doctor.

Beginning date:_____

Day	Medication	BLOOD SUGAR LEVELS						Bedtime	Other
		Breakfast		Lunch		Dinner			
		Before	After*	Before	After*	Before	After*		
Sunday									
Observations									
Monday									
Observations									
Tuesday									
Observations									
Wed.									
Observations									
Thursday									
Observations									
Friday									
Observations									
Saturday									
Observations									

*Take your after-meal readings two hours after the start of the meal.

how to use your blood sugar log

A blood-sugar log is only useful if you look at it, notice patterns, and make adjustments accordingly. Your doctor or certified diabetes educator can help you interpret your log. Use the log in conjunction with the daily food and exercise log on the next page.

Day	Medication	BLOOD SUGAR LEVELS						Bedtime	Other
		Breakfast		Lunch		Dinner			
		Before	After*	Before	After*	Before	After*		
Sunday	Metformin 500mg	80	220						
Observations	Too much carb at breakfast. Tomorrow decrease carbs.								
Monday	Metformin 500mg	92	126						
Observations	80g of carbs at breakfast seems to work better.								
Tuesday	Metformin 500mg	88	122						
Observations	Breakfast carb amount seems okay.								
Wed.	Metformin 500g			118	240				
Observations	Had 3 slices of pizza for lunch!								
Thursday	Metformin 500mg			124	167				
Observations	Ate regular lunch — Sandwich and apple. Better post-lunch levels.								
Friday	Metformin 500mg					111	226		
Observations	After dinner test too high. Too much carb at dinner. Decrease carbs or add exercise.								
Saturday	Metformin 500mg					120	156		
Observations	Decreased carbs to 60 grams but blood sugar still high. Check more pre/post-dinner values next week.								

*Take your after-meal readings two hours after the start of the meal.

daily food and exercise log

Use this chart for a more detailed look at how your meals and physical activity affect your blood sugar. If cutting portion sizes and carbs at one meal still leaves your blood sugar levels high before the next meal, try adding exercise to bring those levels down further.

Day:_____ Date:_____

MORNING

Breakfast Time:_____ Blood sugar before eating:_____

ITEM	AMOUNT	CARBS*

Blood sugar two hours after eating:_____

Snack Time:_____

ITEM	AMOUNT	CARBS*

Exercise Time:_____

ACTIVITY

DURATION

MIDDAY

Lunch Time:_____ Blood sugar before eating:_____

ITEM	AMOUNT	CARBS*

Blood sugar two hours after eating:_____

Snack Time:_____

ITEM	AMOUNT	CARBS*

Exercise Time:_____

ACTIVITY

DURATION

EVENING

Dinner Time:_____ Blood sugar before eating:_____

ITEM	AMOUNT	CARBS*

Blood sugar two hours after eating:_____

Snack Time:_____

ITEM	AMOUNT	CARBS*

Exercise Time:_____

ACTIVITY

DURATION

*choices or grams.

common foods and their glycemic loads

The glycemic load (GL) is a measure of how much a serving of a particular food raises a person's blood sugar. Your own reaction might be somewhat different, so it's smart to check your blood sugar two hours after eating a food to find out how it affects *your* blood sugar. We've grouped foods into three categories: low GL (10 and under), medium GL (11 to 19), and high GL (20 and up). The higher the GL, the more the food will raise your blood sugar.

The GL is closely tied to portion size; if you eat twice as much as the portion size indicated, the food will have double the effect on your blood sugar.

Low (GL = 10 or under)

Breads, Tortillas, Grains	Serving size	GL
Coarse barley bread (75% intact kernels)	2 slices	10
Soy and flaxseed bread	2 slices	10
Whole-grain pumpernickel bread	2 slices	10
Pearled barley	1 cup	8
Popcorn	2 cups	8
Wheat tortillas	2 6-inch	6

Breakfast Cereals	Serving size	GL
Alpen Muesli	⅓ cup (1 oz)	10
Oatmeal, instant	1 cup prepared (1 oz)	10
All-Bran	½ cup (1 oz)	9
Bran Buds	⅓ cup (1 oz)	7
Oatmeal made from rolled oats	1 cup prepared (1 oz)	7

Beans and Peas	Serving size	GL
Lima beans	1 cup	10
Pinto beans	1 cup	10
Chickpeas	1 cup	8
Baked beans	1 cup	7
Kidney beans	1 cup	7
Navy beans	1 cup	7
Butter beans	1 cup	6
Green peas	1 cup	6
Split peas, yellow	1 cup	6
Lentils, green or red	1 cup	5

Dairy and Soy Drinks	Serving size	GL
Low-fat yogurt with fruit and sugar	7 oz	9
Soy milk	1 cup (8 oz)	7
Low-fat chocolate milk, sweetened with aspartame	1 cup (8 oz)	3
Low-fat yogurt with fruit, sweetened with aspartame	7 oz	2

Fruits and Vegetables	Serving size	GL
Prunes, pitted, chopped	⅓ cup (2 oz)	10
Apricots, dried, chopped	⅓ cup (2 oz)	9
Peaches, canned in light syrup	½ cup (4 oz)	9
Grapes, medium bunch (about 50)	4 oz	8
Mango, sliced	⅔ cup (4 oz)	8
Pineapple, diced	⅔ cup (4 oz)	7
Apple	1 small	6
Kiwifruit, sliced	⅔ cup (4 oz)	6
Beets, sliced	½ cup	5
Orange	1 small	5
Peach	1 small	5
Plums	2 small	5
Pear	1 small	4
Strawberries	about 6 medium	4
Watermelon, chopped	⅔ cup (4 oz)	4
Carrots, raw	1 large	3
Cherries	about 16 (4 oz)	3
Grapefruit	½	3

Beverages	Serving size	GL
Orange juice, unsweetened	¾ cup (6 oz)	10
Grapefruit juice, unsweetened	¾ cup (6 oz)	7
Tomato juice	¾ cup (6 oz)	4

Sweets	Serving size	GL
M&Ms with peanuts	25 (1 oz)	6
Nutella (chocolate hazelnut spread)	4 Tbsp	4

Nuts	Serving size	GL
Mixed nuts, roasted	⅓ cup (1.5 oz)	4
Cashew nuts	about 13 (1.5 oz)	3
Peanuts	⅓ cup (1.5 oz)	1

Medium (GL = 11–19)

Bread, Tortillas, Crackers, Chips	Serving size	GL
Coarse barley bread	2 slices	18
High-fiber white bread	2 slices	18
Corn chips	2 oz	17
100% whole-grain bread	2 slices	14
Sourdough rye bread	2 slices	12
Stone-ground wheat thins	4	12
Corn tortillas	2 6-inch	11

Grains	Serving size	GL
Converted long-grain white rice	⅔ cup cooked	16
Brown rice	⅔ cup cooked	18
Quinoa	⅔ cup cooked	16
Wild rice	⅔ cup cooked	18
Wheatberries	⅔ cup cooked	14
Bulgur	⅔ cup cooked	12

Pasta	Serving size	GL
Spaghetti (cooked 15 minutes)	1 cup	17
Whole-wheat spaghetti	1 cup	13
High-protein spaghetti	1 cup	12

Beverages	Serving size	GL
Low-fat chocolate milk	1 cup (8 oz)	12
Pineapple juice, unsweetened	6 oz	12
Apple juice	1 cup (8 oz)	8

Fruits, Vegetables, Beans	Serving size	GL
Sweet corn	1 cup	18
Sweet potato	1 medium (5 oz)	17
Figs, dried, chopped	⅓ cup (2 oz)	16
Banana	1 small (4 oz)	11
Black-eyed peas	1 cup	11

Breakfast Cereals	Serving size	GL
Nabisco Cream of Wheat, regular	1 cup prepared (1 oz)	17
Post Grape-Nuts	½ cup (1 oz)	16
Cheerios	1 cup (1 oz)	15
Life	¾ cup (1 oz)	15
Special K	1 cup (1 oz)	14

High (GL = 20 or higher)

Potatoes	Serving size	GL
Baked white potato	1 medium	26
French fries	5 oz	22

Grains	Serving size	GL
Sticky white rice	⅔ cup cooked	31
Millet	⅔ cup cooked	25
Couscous	⅔ cup cooked	23
Long-grain white rice	⅔ cup cooked	23

Pasta	Serving size	GL
Udon noodles	1 cup cooked	25
Spaghetti (cooked 20 minutes)	1 cup	22

Breads	Serving size	GL
French baguette	2 slices	30
Middle Eastern flatbread	1 large	30
Italian white bread	2 slices	22
Hamburger roll	1	21
Mini-bagel (Lender's)	1	20
Wonder Bread	2 slices	20

Breakfast Cereals	Serving size	GL
Kellogg's Cornflakes	1 cup (1 oz)	24
Rice Chex	1¼ cups (1 oz)	23
Nabisco Cream of Wheat, instant	1 cup prepared (1 oz)	22
Corn Chex	1 cup (1 oz)	21

Dried Fruit	Serving size	GL
Raisins	⅓ cup	28
Dates, dried, chopped	⅓ cup	25

Beverages	Serving size	GL
Cranberry Juice Cocktail	12 oz	36
Coca-Cola	12 oz	24

Sweets	Serving size	GL
Mars Bar	2 oz	26
Jelly beans	20	22
Chocolate cake with chocolate icing	4 oz	20

Source: "International Table of Glycemic Index and Glycemic Load Values 2002," *American Journal of Clinical Nutrition*, vol. 76, no. 1 (2002), 5–56. Additional data from www.glycemicindex.com.

carbohydrate exchanges

One good way to keep your blood sugar under control is to eat approximately the same amount of carbohydrate every day and distribute those carbs fairly evenly throughout the day. Carbohydrate counting helps you do it. Start by knowing how many grams of carbs/"carb choices" you should eat each day (see page 53), then use this list as a handy reference. Each food listed below, in the amount specified, equals approximately 15 grams of carbohydrate (one carb choice) unless otherwise noted. The foods will vary in the number of calories they contain based on their fat and protein content.

One Carb Choice (unless otherwise noted)

Breads
1 slice of bread
¼ large bagel
½ English muffin
1 small muffin
½ hamburger or hot dog bun
6-inch tortilla
⅓ cup stuffing
1 plain small dinner roll
1 waffle
4 Melba toasts

Cereals
½ cup cooked oatmeal or farina
¾ cup dry cereal
1½ cup puffed cereal
½ cup sugar frosted flakes or bran flakes
¼ cup granola

Pastas and Grains
⅓ cup brown or white rice
⅓ cup pasta or other grains, cooked
½ cup chow mein noodles
3 tablespoons flour

Snack-Type Foods
8 animal crackers
3 graham crackers
4 cups of popped popcorn
1 ounce snack chips
6 saltine-type crackers

2 rice cakes
½ cup sugar-free pudding
1 small granola bar
5 vanilla wafers
2 small cookies
½ cup sherbet
½ small cupcake

Vegetables
⅓ cup of cooked dried beans (kidney, pinto, navy)
¼ cup baked beans
½ cup corn, peas
10 french fries
½ cup hash brown potatoes
1 small white or sweet potato
¼ large baked potato
1 cup winter squash
1 cup marinara or tomato-based pasta sauce

Fruits
1 small apple, orange, pear, or peach
7 apricot halves, dried
½ cup unsweetened applesauce
½ banana
1 cup raspberries
⅓ cantaloupe
17 grapes
½ grapefruit
2 tablespoons raisins
1¼ cup strawberries

½ cup fruit juice (apple, orange)
⅓ cup of prune or grape juice
1¼ cup cubed watermelon
1 tablespoon all-fruit jelly or jam

Dairy Foods
1 cup of milk (skim, low-fat, 2%, whole, soy)
½ cup evaporated milk
1 cup plain yogurt
½ cup ice cream or ice milk

Soup
1 cup of cream-based soup (made with water)
1 cup broth-based soup

Sweets (30 grams of carb, or two carb choices)
1 plain doughnut
½ cup regular pudding
1 cup chocolate milk
1 small soft-serve cone

Sweets (45 grams of carb, or three carb choices)
⅙ of a two-crust fruit pie
1 small Danish or sweet roll
1 can (12 ounces) regular soda

Source: The Austin Group, LLC. © 2006.

shopping list

If you're planning your meals as we suggest, create a shopping list based on the recipes on the week's menus. Here's a list of healthy staples to get you started. Remember our advice to fill up to one-half of your shopping cart with colorful produce.

Fresh Foods

Fruit
- ❑ Berries
- ❑ Apples
- ❑ Bananas
- ❑ Oranges or grapefruit
- ❑ Nectarines or peaches
- ❑ Mangoes
- ❑ Kiwifruit
- ❑ Cantaloupe

Protein Foods
- ❑ Fresh fish or seafood
- ❑ Chicken breast
- ❑ Lean beef (limit red meat to two servings per week)
- ❑ Turkey or chicken breast from the deli
- ❑ Eggs

Vegetables
- ❑ Broccoli
- ❑ Spinach
- ❑ Tomatoes (include cherry tomatoes for munching)
- ❑ Carrots (including baby carrots for munching)
- ❑ Shredded carrots for salads
- ❑ Avocado
- ❑ Lettuce (not iceberg)
- ❑ Cabbage or bok choy
- ❑ Red bell peppers
- ❑ Garlic
- ❑ Onions
- ❑ Cauliflower for "cauliflower rice" (page 61)
- ❑ Your veggie of the week

Dairy Counter
- ❑ Skim milk
- ❑ Evaporated skim milk
- ❑ Plain nonfat yogurt
- ❑ Low-fat cheddar or Monterey Jack cheese
- ❑ Low-fat string cheese
- ❑ Feta cheese
- ❑ Soy milk
- ❑ Margarine free of trans fat

Other
- ❑ Flaxseeds, whole
- ❑ Mustard
- ❑ Meal replacement drinks such as Glucerna
- ❑ Hummus (not with tahini)
- ❑ Fresh tomato salsa

Pantry Foods

Grains
- ❑ 100% whole-grain bread
- ❑ Whole-wheat tortillas
- ❑ Whole-wheat pasta
- ❑ Barley
- ❑ Brown rice
- ❑ Old-fashioned oatmeal
- ❑ Couscous (preferably whole-wheat)
- ❑ Cereals with at least 5 grams of fiber per serving

Spices
- ❑ Basil
- ❑ Cayenne
- ❑ Cinnamon

- ❑ Dry rubs for meats
- ❑ Ginger
- ❑ Italian seasoning
- ❑ Lemon-herb seasoning
- ❑ Oregano
- ❑ Rosemary
- ❑ Turmeric (or curry powder)

Canned Goods
- ❑ Water-packed albacore tuna
- ❑ Canned salmon
- ❑ Black, kidney, and pinto beans

Other
- ❑ Extra-virgin olive oil
- ❑ Flaxseed oil
- ❑ Canola oil
- ❑ Walnut oil
- ❑ Natural peanut butter
- ❑ Granola bars with at least 5 gram of fiber and no more than 150 calories per bar
- ❑ Low-fat whole-grain crackers with at least 3 grams of fiber per serving and no trans fats
- ❑ Unsalted nuts
- ❑ 100-calorie snack packs
- ❑ Tea bags
- ❑ Kosher salt

For the Freezer

- ❑ Frozen berries
- ❑ Frozen broccoli florets, carrots, or mixed vegetables
- ❑ Frozen chicken tenderloins
- ❑ Frozen edamame
- ❑ Frozen cod, salmon, or other fish (plain, not breaded)
- ❑ Frozen fish burgers
- ❑ Pre-cleaned shrimp
- ❑ Fruit bars
- ❑ Frozen fudge bars (80 calories each)

sample meal plans

The following menus are examples of just how easy it is to get plenty of fruits and vegetables into your meals and keep calories and carbs under control. Each menu contains approximately 1,600 to 1,800 calories; if you need fewer or more calories per day, you'll need to adjust portion sizes accordingly. Consult your registered dietitian to discuss how these menus might fit into your own eating plan.

Easy Weekday Menu

During the week, everything is a routine. But routine doesn't have to mean boring. Here's an easy, delicious menu for those busy days.

Breakfast
- 1 ounce ready-to-eat high-fiber cereal (5 grams or more per serving)
- 1 cup fat-free milk
- ½ cup fresh blueberries

Lunch
- Honey Mustard Turkey Sandwich: 3 ounces lean turkey breast, 2 slices tomato, 1 lettuce leaf, 2 tablespoons shredded carrots, 2 teaspoons honey mustard, 2 slices (1 ounce each) whole-grain bread
- ¾ cup sliced cucumbers and ½ cup cherry tomatoes drizzled with 1 teaspoon olive oil and 2 teaspoons balsamic vinegar
- 1 Granny Smith apple

Dinner
- 4 ounces broiled tilapia with ⅓ cup *Tropical Fruit Salsa* (page 51)
- ½ cup *Garlicky Green Beans* (page 49)
- ½ cup steamed brown rice
- 1 cup tossed green salad with 2 tablespoons fat-free Italian dressing

Snacks
- ½ cup low-fat cottage cheese sprinkled with ¼ teaspoon pumpkin pie spice
- 1 serving (4 chips) *Crispy Cheese Chips* (page 66)

On the Go

One look at your to-do-list and you know you are going to have one hectic day. Just be prepared with this on-the-go menu that even incorporates a stop at a local fast-food outlet.

Breakfast
- 1 serving *Breakfast Parfait* (page 255) prepared in a portable container
- ½ whole-wheat English muffin spread with 2 teaspoons peanut butter

Lunch
- 1 3.5-ounce plain hamburger from fast-food outlet
- Side salad with low-fat dressing
- 1 small apple (from home if need be)

Dinner
- 1 serving *Fix-It-and-Forget-It Freezer Casserole* (page 41)
- 1 cup tossed green salad with 1 teaspoon olive oil and 2 teaspoons red wine vinegar
- ½ cup fresh pineapple chunks

Snacks
- 1 serving *Garlic-and-Onion Roasted Edamame* (page 206)
- 1 small banana

Weekend

Aaah. The weekend! You've looked forward all week long to putting up your feet and relaxing a bit. Since you have more free time on the weekend, spend a tad more of it in the kitchen whipping up a delectable meal. These menu suggestions require not much more than one pan and just a few extra minutes in the kitchen.

Breakfast

- Egg White Omelet: 3 egg whites mixed with ¼ cup fat-free milk, folded in with ¼ cup chopped red bell pepper and 2 tablespoons minced onion, and cooked in 1 teaspoon non-hydrogenated canola margarine
- 1 slice (1 ounce) whole-wheat toast with 1 teaspoon sugar-free jam
- ½ cup sliced strawberries garnished with 1 orange slice and mint sprig

Lunch

- Sweet Curried Chicken Salad Sandwich: 1 pound cooked diced white chicken, ½ cup diced unpeeled apple, ¼ cup shredded carrots, and 2 tablespoons raisins dressed with ⅓ cup nonfat mayonnaise mixed with 2 teaspoons honey, 1 teaspoon curry powder, and a dash of salt and pepper, served in four whole wheat pita pocket halves and topped with lettuce (makes two sandwiches)
- ½ cup carrot sticks
- 10 red grapes

Dinner

- 1 serving **Balsamic Mustard Grilled Shrimp Kebabs** (page 99)
- ½ cup cooked whole-wheat couscous (serve under the shrimp)
- 1 serving **Apple Coleslaw** (page 97)

Snacks

- 1 serving **Double-Rich Chocolate Pudding Treat** (page 246)
- 1 small peach

Company's Coming

Everyone will enjoy this special menu whether they have diabetes or not. In fact, expect your guests will want another invite soon.

Breakfast

- 1 frozen whole-grain waffle
- 2 teaspoons sugar-free maple syrup
- ½ cup raspberries
- 1 cup fat-free milk

Lunch

- 1 serving **Barley and Chickpea Salad** (page 21)
- 1 cup romaine lettuce tossed with ¼ cup diced cucumbers and ¼ cup shredded carrots drizzled with 1 teaspoon walnut oil and 2 teaspoons herb vinegar
- 1 small nectarine

Dinner

- 1 serving **Seared Cod in Zesty Herb and Tomato Sauce** (page 224)
- ½ cup steamed broccoli or broccolini
- ½ cup whole-wheat penne noodles

Snacks

- 1 serving **Sweet Balsamic Onion and White Bean Spread** (page 70) with 1 ounce whole-wheat crackers
- ¼ sliced mango sprinkled with 1 teaspoon lime juice

handy numbers to know

General Blood Sugar Targets

Fasting or before meal glucose	90–130 mg/dl
After-meal glucose (two hours after the start of your meal)	>180 mg/dl
Bedtime glucose	100–140 mg/dl

How to Translate A1C Numbers

A1C	Blood Glucose Level	
6.0%	135 mg/dl	7.5 mmol/l*
6.5%	153 mg/dl	8.5 mmol/l*
7.0%	170 mg/dl	9.5 mmol/l*
7.5%	188 mg/dl	10.5 mmol/l*
8.0%	205 mg/dl	11.4 mmol/l*
8.5%	223 mg/dl	12.4 mmol/l*
9.0%	240 mg/dl	13.3 mmol/l*
9.5%	258 mg/dl	14.3 mmol/l*
10.0%	275 mg/dl	15.3 mmol/l*
10.5%	293 mg/dl	16.3 mmol/l*
11.0%	310 mg/dl	17.2 mmol/l*
11.5%	328 mg/dl	18.2 mmol/l*
12.0%	345 mg/dl	19.1 mmol/l*

* Millimoles per liter, used outside the U.S.

Healthy Waist Circumference

Men	up to 40 inches
Women	up to 35 inches

If your waist is bigger than this, you are at increased risk for type 2 diabetes, high blood pressure, high cholesterol, and cardiovascular disease.

index